Dental Law and Ethics

Edited by
Paul Lambden

Radcliffe Medical Press

Radcliffe Medical Press Ltd
18 Marcham Road
Abingdon
Oxon OX14 1AA
United Kingdom

www.radcliffe-oxford.com
The Radcliffe Medical Press electronic catalogue and online ordering facility.
Direct sales to anywhere in the world.

British Library Cataloguing in Publication Data

A catalogue record for this book is available from the British Library.

ISBN 1 85775 911 7

Typeset by Aarontype Limited, Easton, Bristol
Printed and bound by TJ International Ltd, Padstow, Cornwall

Contents

Preface

Ethics is the science of the morals of human conduct and provides the principles that rule the behaviour of society. The law is the enactment of custom or statute which is recognised as permitting or prohibiting certain actions and which is enforced by the imposition of penalties. The common strand that links ethics and law is that it provides the standard expected by society, identified by the former and upheld by the latter.

Ethical principles are integral to the dental profession. The General Dental Council makes clear that all dentists should maintain the highest ethical standards and it is against them that their conduct will be judged. Recent high-profile cases have highlighted situations where the behaviour and actions of dentists have fallen below that expected by the profession as a whole and the changes embodied in revalidation and continuing education combined with clear guidance on practice standards reaffirm and strengthen the values to which all practitioners should aspire.

Ethical guidance should be positive, demonstrating best practice and providing guidance on the appropriate standards of personal and professional behaviour. Those practitioners whose actions or conduct fall below the expected standard dishonour not only themselves but the profession as a whole. Such actions open them to allegations of professional misconduct which may in turn result in the loss of their livelihood, their professional standing in the community and considerable damage to personal and professional relationships. However, maintenance of standards should not be regarded as a burden. It is merely the exercise of what is to be expected from reasonable people under normal circumstances. Without it the profession could not flourish in the way that it has done.

This book will be invaluable to students and practitioners alike. Its chapters have been written by a wide range of distinguished contributors who, between them, have expertise in a wide range of aspects of dental practice. Their contributions are very readable yet authoritative. The book addresses the key areas of practice where legal and ethical issues have an impact on day-to-day practice. Subjects include consent and confidentiality, complaints and negligence, as well as tackling the more difficult problems such as those associated with patients who are mentally disabled and therefore not able to protect their own rights and freedoms. There is also a chapter on the workings of the General Dental Council and a review of the work of the Dental Practice Board.

Each chapter is complete on its own and can be read individually or as part of the overall subject matter. For that reason there is some duplication within some of the chapters. This was done deliberately to make for simpler reading rather than requiring the reader to refer back to other parts of the book. It has also allowed the individual authors to express their own perspectives on some of the more crucial elements of law and ethics.

Bertrand Russell said: 'Man is not a solitary animal, and so long as social life survives, self-realisation cannot be the supreme principle of ethics'. Dentistry, as part of healthcare, is at the centre of the fabric of society. Ethics and law cannot be ignored and, for that reason, this book is essential reading for every undergraduate and every dental healthcare professional.

Dr Paul Lambden
Medical and Dental Principal
St. Paul International Insurance Company
November 2001

About the editor

Dr Paul Lambden BSc MB BS BDS FDSRCS MRCS LRCP DRCOG MHSM
Paul Lambden graduated in medicine, dentistry and science at Guy's Hospital, London. After working initially in oral medicine and surgery and gaining his Fellowship of the Royal College of Surgeons of England, he entered general medical and dental practice, continuing the two for 15 years.

During his time in primary care he worked part-time as a clinical tutor at St. Bartholomew's Hospital, London. He was an enthusiastic first wave GP fundholder.

In 1992 he left general practice to become the Chief Executive of a whole district NHS Trust and also worked as a special adviser to the all-party Parliamentary Health Select Committee. He subsequently went on to become the Chairman and Chief Executive of a charity and is now the Medical and Dental Principal of St. Paul International Insurance Company Ltd.

Paul is a regular writer on medical, health and management topics. He has appeared on many radio and television programmes and recently completed a series of programmes for a medical television channel.

About the contributors

Andrew Bridgman

Andrew Bridgman, exiled from Wales since 1976, qualified in dentistry from the Turner Dental School, Manchester, in 1981. He became a partner in a well-established south Manchester practice in 1989 and, in keeping with the tradition at that practice, became a part-time clinical teacher in Restorative Dentistry at his alma mater. At the same time, he embarked upon part-time study for a Law degree and graduated in 1994. A serious rugby injury enforced retirement from general practice in 1995. Having held the additional appointment of Lecturer in Ethics and Law for Dentistry since 1992 he decided to develop his interest in ethics and the law relating to healthcare and undertook further study, gaining an MA (Health Care Ethics and Law) in 1998.

Andrew Collier

Andrew Collier is a clinical teacher in the Restorative Department of Leeds Dental School, where he also runs the course in General Dental Practice.

Andrew is a dento-legal adviser for Dental Protection. He has a particular interest in team working and in dental team training. He is also a dental nurse examiner and postgraduate dental tutor for Leeds.

David Corless-Smith

David Corless-Smith is a solicitor and dentist and partner at the Dental Law Partnership, a firm of solicitors specialising in dental negligence litigation.

Christopher Dean

Chris Dean has been a practising general dental practitioner since 1985. He has a Law degree, an MA in medical ethics and law and was called to the Bar in 1999. He is also the Managing Director of the Dental Law Company, which provides clinical case screening services for patients in dental negligence claims.

David E Gibbons
David Gibbons is Newland-Pedley Professor of Oral Health Services Research, Head of Department and Consultant in Dental Public Health at Guy's, King's and St Thomas' Dental Institute of King's College, London. He has responsibility for the teaching of dental ethics both in the under- graduate curriculum and in the common core course for postgraduates undertaking MScs and PhDs.

He has been a member of a Multicentre Research Ethics Committee (MREC) for several years. His career has spanned general dental practice, management of community dental services, dental public health and for four years, he left dentistry to become a health authority general manager.

Helen Kaney
Helen Kaney works within the Professional Services Team-Healthcare as a dento-legal adviser and advises and supports The St. Paul policyholders on all dento-legal matters arising from their clinical practice.

Helen qualified in dentistry from Glasgow University in 1987 and worked as an NHS general dental practitioner in the west of Scotland until December 1998. She completed a Law degree in 1997 and also works as an honorary clinical demonstrator in the Department of Conservative Dentistry at Guy's Dental Hospital.

Jenny King
Jenny King teaches ethics and law to dental students at Bart's and the London School of Medicine and Dentistry at Queen Mary College, London University. Her current research interests are the practicalities of consent in the dental surgery and the moral importance of respect for personal autonomy. She is a theologian and dentist and for many years taught chil- dren's dentistry.

Margaret Seward
Dame Margaret Seward is the Chief Dental Officer for England at the Depart- ment of Health. She was the first woman to be elected to the General Dental Council, becoming its President in 1994 for a five-year term. She was also President of the Dental Association from 1993 to 1994.

Dame Margaret qualified at the London Hospital Dental School and special- ised in oral surgery. She became full-time Editor of the *British Dental Journal* in 1978 and Editor of the *International Dental Journal* in 1989. A leading figure in the Federation Dentaire Internationale, she has chaired its Commu- nications and Ethics and Legislation committees and served on its Council from 1989 to 1992.

Dame Margaret has lectured extensively at home and abroad, written numerous leaders and articles in the national and international press and was Director for Teamwork from 1990 to 2000. She is currently the Director of the 'Better Opportunities for Women Dentists' project, aimed at improving career aspirations and commitment to the workforce.

She has been recognised nationally with awards of honorary doctorates from universities, honorary fellowships from the Surgical Royal Colleges and honorary membership of specialised societies. Internationally, she is an invited honorary member of the Pierre Fauchard Academy, the International College of Dentists and the College of Dental Surgeons in Hong Kong.

Amolak Singh

Amolak Singh has been a general dental practitioner for 40 years. He obtained a Diploma in Medical Ethics and Law from King's College, University of London, in 1985 followed by a Law degree (LLB) in 1987.

He has been an elected member of the General Dental Council since 1991, a member of the General Dental Services Committee for the past 10 years and also a member of its Statutes and Regulations Subcommittee.

He is Chief Executive of the GDPA, a former President of the Anglo Asian Odontological Group and was a member of the BUPA Dental Advisory Panel from 1992 to 1997. He was Chairman of the Council of Managerial and Professional Staffs, the UK's largest independent trade union, from 1994 to 1997 and is presently a member of its Executive Committee.

Amolak Singh was appointed by the Secretary of State as a member of the Employment Tribunals (England and Wales) in 1992 and to the Criminal Injuries Compensation Appeals Panel in 1996.

Greg Waldron

Greg Waldron qualified as a dentist in 1986 and as a solicitor in 1997. He is a partner in the Dental Law Partnership and Chairman of the Dental Law Company which acts on behalf of dental patients in the UK.

He is the Founding Secretary of the UK Dental Law and Ethics Forum, Founding Treasurer of the International Dental Ethics and Law Society and author of various articles in the UK dental press.

Graham Walsh

Graham Walsh BChD LDS (Leeds) graduated in 1966, and for 20 years practised in the Huddersfield area. He took a law degree and was called to the bar in 1992 (Inner Temple). For the last 16 years he has worked as a Dental Reference Officer, first with the Department of Health, and since 1990, with the Dental Practice Board. He was promoted to Senior Dental Officer in 1998. Graham was recently awarded the Diploma in Advanced Litigation from Nottingham Law School and is hoping to complete the LLM degree in June 2002.

Acknowledgement

This book would not have been possible without the generous support of St. Paul International Insurance Company. It was conceived, developed and completed with their support and the company has had the vision to see the value and merit of such a book and provide the funding for the first edition.

Further acknowledgements

This book is the result of an enormous amount of hard work on the part of the contributors. They have all very generously agreed that all royalties from this book will go to charity.

I am particularly grateful to Dr Jenny King, Lecturer in Law and Ethics at the St. Bartholomew's and The Royal London School of Medicine and Dentistry, and to Mr Andrew Bridgman, Lecturer at the University Dental Hospital of Manchester, for the considerable time they have spent in reviewing the chapters and constructing the format of the book. The difficulty of arranging the chapters into a readable and convenient layout cannot be overstated.

Also to Helen King who has worked tirelessly to get the 14 disparate chapters into a consistent style and layout.

Finally to Greg Waldron whose original idea this book actually was. He spent a considerable amount of his own time recruiting the contributors and the effort he put into the book has been much appreciated.

CHAPTER ONE

The General Dental Council

Margaret Seward

Quality and standards are at the very heart of the activities of a professional regulatory body and for the dental profession that body is the General Dental Council (GDC). It is often stated that professional self-regulation is a bargain or a contract between the profession and the state for the maintenance of the highest standards of care and for the protection of the public. Any such regulatory process is a privilege and in return there needs to be accountability, consistency and transparency in all its actions and activities. At the same time, any regulatory mechanism, which in this case is financed solely by the members of the profession through the payment of an annual fee, should also be seen as one which supports the highest ethical principles of the professional group which it represents.

Principles of regulation

While the primary focus of the statutory regulatory process is to protect the public there is no doubt that it does have other advantages. First, it enhances the status of the profession and second, it provides some assurance of the standards of the professionals in the working environment. This is achieved through either published ethical guidance or the inspection of undergraduate courses as provided by dental schools or faculties, ensuring the highest standards of educational provisions are met.

However, there remain certain common misunderstandings about professional regulation in general terms. It cannot and should not be used as a substitute for the well-established systems of civil redress. The actions normally taken by regulatory bodies are, to put it simply, to protect a member of the public, a patient, from a professional, a dentist, hygienist or therapist, who may either cause him/her harm or undertake treatment which falls short of the expected standards which would have been provided by their peers. The self-regulatory process is certainly not designed to award compensation to the affected parties and again, it is certainly not a substitute for a matter of concern, for example fraud, which clearly needs to be investigated by the police or criminal courts who then decide on the appropriate punishment or penalty.

It is important to remember that the GDC does not aim to punish dentists and when a dentist's name is removed from the Dentists Register following an inquiry, this action is taken solely to protect the public. However, this is often wrongly seen as a punishment because the dentist, as a consequence of being 'struck off', is deprived of his or her livelihood.

Another common area of doubt relating to the activities of the GDC is in relation to employment matters. Effective management is for employees and employers to work out together.

Any professional regulatory system can only work satisfactorily and retain public confidence if the members of the profession adhere to the highest ethical principles. 'Do as you would be done by' when dealing with members of the public or, to be specific, patients is the sure maxim to gain success.

The Council and its composition

The General Dental Council was established in 1956 by a Dentists Act, so creating an independent profession. Before this time the General Medical Council held overall responsibility for dentistry, although the business was administered by the Dental Board of the United Kingdom which was established by the Dentists Act of 1921.

At the present time the General Dental Council operates in line with the current legislation which is contained within the 1984 Dentists Act.[1] Repeated efforts have been made by the profession since 1992 for changes to the primary legislation, but so far have not met with success. However, the Health Act 1999[2] included Order Making Powers, which it is hoped will facilitate the much-needed reforms to specific areas of current legislation. These, for example, could allow the introduction of mandatory recertification for all dentists, increase the number of lay people on the Council, permit the establishment of poor performance procedures and the statutory registration of all Professionals Complementary to Dentistry (PCD). This would mean that dental nurses and dental technicians would join the dental hygienists and dental therapists who are currently registered with the Council.

The mission of the GDC clearly states that it is the regulatory body of the dental profession; it protects the public by means of its statutory responsibilities for dental education, registration, professional conduct and health.

It also states that it supports dentists and dental auxiliaries (PCDs) in the practice of dentistry and encourages their continuing professional development.

The Council has 50 members who elect the President from amongst its number for a term of five years. The remaining 18 dentists on the Council come from four designated constituencies in the UK but they represent the whole profession: England, Isle of Man and the Channel Islands elects 14 members, Scotland elects two members, Wales and Northern Ireland one member each.

A further 17 members are nominated by the dental authorities who award the qualifying degrees and diplomas such as the universities with dental schools and the Surgical Royal Colleges which have dental faculties. There are six lay members appointed by the Privy Council and four Chief Dental Officers, again representing the four constituencies – England, Scotland, Wales and Northern Ireland. Maintaining the historical link with the General Medical Council, three members are doctors who are also members of the GMC and are nominated to serve on the GDC. As a consequence of the 1984 Dentists Act, one dental auxiliary can sit on the full Council and is elected by the Dental Auxiliaries Committee of the GDC.

The term of office for all members is five years but the election of the dentists and the nomination of appointed members does not take place concurrently, so permitting stability and continuity of the Council's work. On 1 October 1999, the President and 17 nominated members began a new five-year term of office and the most recent election of dentists and the one auxiliary member was held in May 2001. The successful candidates took office on 1 October 2001. There is a new electoral system in operation which replaced the former and complicated system of the single transferable vote (STV). In addition there has been a reorganisation of the constituencies to allow for national and regional candidates to be elected, so improving understanding of the activities of the statutory regulatory body among members of the profession and also encouraging them to participate in the quinquennial elections.

The major activities of the Council, that is registration, education, conduct and health and dental auxiliaries (PCDs), are conducted through committees on which members of the Council serve. The composition and procedures of each committee are determined by regulations and schedules contained within the Dentists Act 1984.

However, in order to permit more speedy consideration of single and important issues review groups are set up to prepare documents for consultation and report. Topics considered by review groups in the past few years have included general professional training, general anaesthesia and sedation, specialist registration, recertification, postgraduate visitations and a new international qualification.

Registration

Dentists who want to practise dentistry in the UK must have their name on the Dentists Register, for which they pay an annual amount of money called the 'retention fee'. There is no provision in the Dentists Act to allow a reduced rate for either a part-time practitioner or someone who takes a career break from dentistry, but a practitioner over 65 can apply for the 'retired practitioner's rate'.

There are two categories of registration: full and temporary. Those entitled to full registration are graduates or licentiates of UK dental authorities, holders of recognised overseas diplomas, nationals of EU member states who are holders of recognised European diplomas and overseas dentists successful in the Council's statutory examination or from universities abroad whose undergraduate course has been recognised by the GDC.

In fact, the arrangements for entry of graduates from overseas universities changed in 2001. The statutory examination has been replaced by a new examination called the International Qualifying Examination (IQE) which must be taken by all overseas graduates wishing to practise in the UK. This also applies to those dentists graduating after 2001 from previously recognised universities abroad, such as in Australia, South Africa and Malaysia. As a consequence the traditional visitations undertaken by the Council to overseas universities to inspect their dental courses will be discontinued.

The second category, temporary registration, is to allow dentists from overseas to work for a maximum period of four years in the UK in order to undertake teaching, research or postgraduate study for an additional degree or diploma. Those dentists who hold temporary registration can only work in a dental school or an NHS hospital or other institute in a post approved for training by one of the Surgical Royal Colleges of the UK or for research or teaching in a specified and approved position. A dentist with temporary registration is not permitted to work in a general dental practice.

Auxiliaries

All dental hygienists and dental therapists who possess a UK diploma in dental hygiene or dental therapy can ask to have their names entered on the Rolls of Dental Auxiliaries, which is published annually by the GDC. In common with dentists, each auxiliary has to pay a retention fee each year, although at a lower rate, and anyone who practises dentistry without being registered is working illegally and can be prosecuted. Hygienists or therapists qualified in the EU can gain entry to the UK Roll.

Specialists

Since 1998 recognised specialists in a distinctive branch of dentistry can apply for their name to be entered on the appropriate specialist list on the payment of an additional annual fee. This was provided for by the respective European and Primary Specialist Dental Regulations and the GDC's own Domestic Regulations for Specialists passed in 1998. The specialists' lists are currently in dental public health, endodontics, oral surgery, orthodontics, paediatric dentistry, periodontics, prosthodontics, restorative dentistry and surgical dentistry.

A unique document in connection with specialist training, called 'the Accord', was originated by the GDC in 1996. This agreement details the partnership between the GDC, the faculties of dental surgery, the specialist societies, the universities, the postgraduate dental deans and directors and the Joint Committee for Specialist Training in Dentistry.

The educational continuum

The Council ensures the highest standards of education throughout the lifetime of a dentist. Section (1)2 of the 1984 Dentists Act states: 'It shall be the general concern of the Council to promote high standards of dental education at all its stages ...'. This encompasses undergraduate vocational training, general professional training and continuing professional development. This is referred to as the continuum of dental education.

The First Five Years[3] published by the Council, states the requirements of the undergraduate course and visitors are appointed by the GDC to ensure that the course of instruction at the dental school, as well as the qualifying examination, meet the expected standards. The satisfactory outcome of the dental undergraduate course is to produce a dentist who is able to practise independently without supervision.

The introduction of mandatory vocational training in 1995 for dentists who enter NHS dental practice provides the new graduate with a protected environment in which to work for one year with a senior practitioner who is appointed as a vocational trainer.

For a professional, lifelong learning is no longer an option but an obligation. In April 2000 a preparatory scheme for recertification of dentists on a five-year cycle was launched as a prelude to a compulsory scheme, which will be possible when the Dentists Act 1984 is amended by an Order Making Power contained in the Health Act 1999. The aim of recertification is to demonstrate that dentists whose names appear on the Dentists Register have undertaken regular continuing dental education, so showing a commitment to keep up to date in order to maintain competence.

Although the GDC has legal powers to visit and approve all postgraduate degrees, diplomas and courses, it has so far only exercised its right in relation to postgraduate degrees and diplomas from universities and Royal Colleges and has not sought to give approval to courses run by postgraduate deaneries or by commercial organisations.

The curricula for the various distinctive branches of specialist training are approved by the Council through its Specialist Training Advisory Committee, which has representatives in its membership from various professional bodies, as well as the three deans of the dental faculties of the Surgical Royal Colleges.

Curricula are also published by the GDC for the courses in dental therapy and dental hygiene.[4] Training for the diplomas in this subject has traditionally taken place within university dental schools. However, recently training courses have been established outside these recognised venues and qualifying examinations have been established through the surgical Royal Colleges and their faculties. A dental hygienist works in all branches of dentistry but a dental therapist is only permitted to work in dental departments of NHS hospitals or in community dental clinics. Some schools for dental auxiliaries run a combined course so that a student qualifies after two and a half years as a therapist as well as a hygienist. All courses and examinations for auxiliaries are approved in the same way as the undergraduate courses for dentists, by appointing visitors from the GDC to assess the course and examination. Auxiliaries are now known as Professionals Complementary to Dentistry (PCD) and have a similar ethical obligation to keep up to date and maintain competence throughout their practising lifetime.

Professional standards

Section (1)2 of the 1984 Dentists Act states: 'It shall be the concern of the Council to promote high standards of professional conduct among dentists ...' and this is a vitally supportive role in protecting the public.

Maintaining standards

Dentists enjoy the privilege of self-regulation and with that comes the responsibility to maintain the highest standards of ethical dental practice.

The demands of dental practice on practitioners in all disciplines are recognised but dentists should at all times act reasonably and in the public interest. While the Dentists Act states the law, the guidance to dentists on professional and personal conduct covers identified areas of practice where experience suggests that there might be potential for problems to arise which in many instances might have been avoided if the necessary precautions had been taken at the outset. The ethical guidance entitled *Maintaining Standards*,[5] first published in November 1997, aims to be positive and focuses on best practice rather than conduct, which can lead to disciplinary action. The guidance is published in an A4 ring binder format to facilitate the filing of new updated guide sheets published on a regular basis. The contents of the ethical guidance are clearly structured, giving important advice on steps to be taken before beginning to practise: what the public expects; what the patient expects and information on the dental team and practice arrangements as well as information on the Council's jurisdiction.

Conduct procedures

The Council maintains professional standards of dentists and PCDs not only by issuing guidelines but also by the use of its various disciplinary powers, which are given to the GDC under the 1984 Dentists Act.

Preliminary screener

The President, as preliminary screener, receives reports of criminal convictions from the police or complaints from patients as well as from other sources, which might be an officer of a health authority, health board, NHS trust or similar public bodies. Since May 2000, a complaint from a member of the public need not be supported by a legal document such as a statutory declaration or an affidavit which is designed to make it easier for patients to access the complaints process. Advice on how to complain is provided in a leaflet published by the GDC.[6]

The President has to consider whether the complaint or conviction provides *prima facie* evidence of serious professional misconduct. This is defined by the Judicial Committee of the Privy Council in 1987 as conduct connected with his/her profession in which the dentist concerned has fallen short, by omission or commission, of the standards of conduct expected among dentists and that such falling short as is established should be serious? This is the only charge that can be brought against a member of the dental team. If the President decides that there is no case to answer the complainant will be informed and this is the end of the matter. If the

President believes that there may be a case to answer and further information or investigation is required, it will be referred to the Preliminary
Proceedings Committee.

Preliminary Proceedings Committee

When the decision has been taken to refer the matter to the Preliminary
Proceedings Committee (PPC) the dentist will be told and invited to submit
his or her comments or observations on the complaint. These are normally
submitted by the dentist's defence organisation on his or her behalf,
although legally the dentist can respond directly on his or her own account.

The PPC, which normally meets twice a year in March and September,
will consider the complaint and any written response from the dentist
giving explanations for his/her action. The Committee may decide that
there is no case of serious professional misconduct to answer and so the
matter does not proceed and the interested parties are told of this outcome.

Alternatively the Committee may decide that the case is sufficiently
serious or there is enough evidence to suggest that serious professional misconduct may have taken place and that in the interest of public safety the
case must continue. They will then refer the complaint for an inquiry by
the Professional Conduct Committee (PCC) which sits in public normally
twice a year, in May and November, although recently additional hearings
have been held in January, August and September, due to an increase in the
number of cases under consideration.

If it is believed that it is necessary to protect the public at once, then a
meeting of the PPC will be held with the dentist in attendance and legally
represented to consider suspension of the dentist's registration with
immediate effect, which is officially referred to as interim suspension until
the matter is considered by the full Professional Conduct Committee.

On the other hand, the Committee may decide that the matter under consideration does not amount to serious professional misconduct but the
conduct of the dentist as a professional still causes concern. A letter of
advice can be sent to the dentist as a warning of varying severity. This will
then conclude the matter although this information will be taken into
account if further similar complaints against the practitioner arise.

Professional Conduct Committee

The Professional Conduct Committee (PCC) meets in public and consists of
11 Council members. Two are lay members and of the remaining nine

members, at least five must be elected Council members. Advice on all matters of law and procedure is given by a legal assessor who is a senior barrister. The sessions take place in the Council chamber at the headquarters of the Council in Wimpole Street and members of the press and public are able to attend. During the last two years there has been a substantial increase in the number of cases referred to the Council and the subsequent activity of its disciplinary committees. In the 1980s the public hearings of the PCC took place normally in May and September and lasted for 5–6 days. In the 1990s the workload increased and the May and September sessions usually lasted for 8–10 days. In 1999 there was a further increase to five sessions of the PCC, amounting to a total of 35 days, and this number was again exceeded in 2000.

Table 1.1 Professional Conduct Committee. Number of cases heard during the last five years and their determination

	Cases heard	Erasure and suspension
1995	11	4
1996	13	7
1997	14	8
1998	21	5
1999	20	11

The President or his/her appointed representative chairs the hearing, which follows the procedure as for any UK Court, including rules of evidence, sworn statements and witnesses giving testimony under oath. A barrister or solicitor acts on behalf of the GDC and normally the dentist charged with serious professional misconduct will be similarly represented by a barrister or solicitor through a defence organisation. In conduct cases the Committee must first decide whether the facts alleged in the charge are proved. The standard of proof is the same as in a criminal court, namely 'beyond reasonable doubt'. If the facts are found proved the Committee has then to decide whether or not these amount to serious professional misconduct.

The Committee considers a wide range of allegations.

Example 1
A dentist failed to submit forms FP17A for prior approval of treatment and to submit clinical records to the Board. He was found guilty of serious professional misconduct because he did not comply with the NHS Regulations with which he was contracted.

Example 2

In another case, serious consequences arose during the administration of a dental anaesthetic and raised fundamental issues about the relative responsibilities of the professionally qualified dental staff involved in giving general anaesthesia in dentistry. The GDC received its guidance and subsequently amended *Maintaining Standards*[5] to indicate that dentists are no longer permitted to administer a general anaesthetic.

Example 3

Another case involved allegations that a dentist proposed and carried out dental treatment that was not clinically necessary and, in some cases, not appropriate. He was also accused of failure to provide treatment plans and estimates of the cost of the proposed treatment. Further, he allegedly failed to explain the nature of the contract to the patient or act in the best interests of the patient by failing to exercise a proper degree of skill and attention and providing postoperative dental care and treatment. The dentist was found guilty of serious professional misconduct and his name was erased from the Register with immediate effect.

Example 4

Another dentist was found guilty of serious professional misconduct and her registration was suspended for six months after she demanded and received private fees to which she was not entitled as she was treating the patient under existing NHS regulations.

Example 5

An orthodontist was found guilty of serious professional misconduct after making fraudulent claims for orthodontic treatment not undertaken as well as for deliberately damaging orthodontic appliances to make claims for an additional fee for repairs.

Example 6

A dentist was charged with instructing dental nurses to take impressions of patients' mouths and to fix orthodontic brackets. Such procedures amounted to the illegal practice of dentistry by unregistered auxiliary members and the dentist was found guilty of covering, which led to him being found guilty of serious professional misconduct and erasure from the Register.

Example 7

A dentist, disqualified from driving due to excess alcohol over the limit, was reported to the GDC following a motoring offence. He then further drove the car while disqualified and not insured and was involved in a traffic accident. This was a standard of conduct unacceptable from a professional person and his name was erased from the Register.

Where the dentist has already been convicted in a criminal court or found guilty of serious professional misconduct, there are a number of options open to the Committee for the conclusion or disposal of the case. These are: to postpone a final decision, usually for one year, pending reports on the dentist's progress in the meantime; to give an admonition to the dentist; to suspend the dentist's registration for a period of time, for example up to one year; or to strike off or erase the dentist's name from the Register, which is the ultimate sanction.

A dentist who is suspended or erased from the Register has the right to appeal to the Judicial Committee of the Privy Council. In either circumstance, the decision of the PCC does not take effect until 28 days have elapsed. An exception to this is if the Committee feels that there is an urgent need to protect the public in which case the dentist's registration can be suspended with immediate effect. When the senior judges who comprise the Privy Council hear an appeal they will not usually pronounce on professional matters, but on possible miscarriage of justice as seen through the procedures of the case. It is gratifying to note that it is very rare for an appeal to be successful.

Health Committee

Following the 1984 Dentists Act the Council was able to establish a Health Committee. This enables the GDC to consider dentists whose fitness to practise may be seriously impaired because of a physical or mental illness. Most of the cases considered relate to alcohol or drug abuse.

The hearings before the Health Committee are held *in camera* in a sympathetic atmosphere with a non-confrontational procedure. Again, the composition of the Committee is stipulated by the Act and it is chaired by a senior member of the Council who is assisted by a legal assessor and has additionally two medical assessors to advise the Committee on the medical conditions as appropriate.

If the Committee decides that a dentist's fitness to practise is seriously impaired, it may either suspend or impose conditions on his or her registration. Such conditions may include, for example, not working in a single-handed dental practice or undertaking a certain clinical procedure. Suspension and conditions on practice are reviewed at regular intervals. The conditional registration usually also entails certain medical supervision and the support of a professional colleague. By means of these procedures sick dentists are allowed to continue practising in dentistry with adequate support mechanisms in place, which protect the public.

Key role

In the interests of the protection of the public, the General Dental Council, as the self-governing and regulatory body of the dental profession, must maintain the key role of preserving at all times the highest professional standards in pursuit of the quality of care which must be provided for the benefit of all patients.

References and notes

1 Dentists Act 1984. HMSO, London.
2 Health Act 1999. HMSO, London.
3 General Dental Council (1997) *The First Five Years*. GDC, London.
4 General Dental Council (1998) *Curricula for Dental Hygienists and Dental Therapists*. GDC, London.
5 General Dental Council (1997) *Maintaining Standards: guidance to dentists on professional and personal conduct*. GDC, London.
6 General Dental Council (1999) *Complaint and Discipline Procedures: a guide for health authorities, health boards and NHS trusts*. GDC, London.

CHAPTER TWO

Rights and responsibilities in dentistry

Jenny King

> Covenant fidelity is the inner meaning and purpose of our creation as human beings.
>
> *(Paul Ramsey, in the preface to The Patient as Person)*

Dental diseases are common and few people can escape the need for treatment at some time in their lives. Dentistry in western countries has become a well-established profession providing dental care to individuals and communities. Not only can much be done to alleviate pain and infection and restore function and appearance but over recent decades there has been considerable progress in preventing dental disease. Dentists may not often consciously reflect on the ethical and legal principles on which their professional practice is based and yet dentists must make moral judgements throughout the working day. In conduct, in relationships and in decision making good professional practice depends on the expectation by both the profession and the public that dentists work to the highest moral and legal standards. When a person agrees to have dental care two people enter into a moral relationship which is based on mutual obligations. The purpose of this book is to explore the ethical and legal framework in which the provision of healthcare – including dental care – operates. This chapter begins by considering the rights and the responsibilities of those who receive and those who provide healthcare.

Human rights and healthcare

The United Nations Declaration in 1948[1] was an important document which articulated fundamental human rights and has been the basis for much of the development of common moral and legal standards in the second half of the 20th century. These rights were recognised by the Declaration as being universal.

Article 25 states that:

> Everyone has a right to a standard of living adequate for the health and well-being of himself and his family, including food, clothing, housing and medical care and necessary social services.

Since then debates have recognised the rights of vulnerable groups such as women[2] and children.[3]

International human rights law is of increasing significance and the establishment of the European Court of Human Rights has been a further important development.[4] The European Convention and the Human Rights Act[5] can be expected to have a considerable impact on national jurisdiction and in medical law in the future. This includes the right to life and protection from inhuman or degrading treatment. These developments mark a slow but definite shift from the earlier emphasis on professional obligations towards a new emphasis on patients' rights.[6]

The foundation for the British National Health Service was also set up in the 1940s in the aftermath of the Second World War. The establishment of the National Health Service honoured the right to healthcare.[4] It was based on healthcare being available, free at the point of delivery and for all. This includes the provision of dental treatment. There have been many changes since the start of the National Health Service, for example, dental care is now no longer free of any charge to all patients, but the founding principle of the right of everyone to a high standard of healthcare remains.

Dentists' and patients' rights and responsibilities

More recently in 1995 the rights of patients were set out in the Patient's Charter for the NHS.[7] The Charter includes the right to be given information and to have any proposed treatment, including any risks involved in that treatment and any alternatives, clearly explained before deciding whether to agree to it. Patients can expect privacy and NHS staff have a legal duty to keep medical records confidential. Patients registered with a dentist have a right to emergency care.

Medicine and dentistry are governed by statutory self-regulating bodies. In dentistry and complementary professions the General Dental Council must ensure the high ethical and legal standards of the dental profession. It has a duty to keep a register of dentists and oversee dental education and dental practitioners' conduct.

The details of a dentist's responsibilities are set out in the Council's publication *Maintaining Standards*.[8] Dentists have a responsibility to always act in the patient's best interest and provide the highest standards of clinical care. They have a duty to ensure confidentiality and patients' consent to treatment. Failure to follow the General Dental Council guidelines can result in a charge of serious professional misconduct and erasure from the dental list.

Duties of a dentist[9]

The GDC requires every dentist to affirm that:

As a member of the dental profession I will:

- make the care of my patients my first concern, treat every patient politely and considerately, and have respect for patients' dignity and privacy
- listen to patients and respect their views and give patients information in a way which they can understand
- respect the rights of patients to be involved fully in decisions about their care
- make sure that my personal beliefs do not prejudice my patients' care
- act quickly to protect patients from risks if I have good reason to believe that I or a colleague may not be fit to practise
- keep my professional knowledge and skills up to date and recognise the limits of my professional competence
- be honest and trustworthy and respect and protect confidential infor-
- mation
- never discriminate unfairly against my patients or colleagues and be prepared always to justify my actions to them
- avoid abusing my position as a member of the dental profession and work with colleagues in ways which best serve patients' interests.

Not only do dentists have responsibilities towards individual patients but the dental profession also has public health responsibilities to the community,[10] for example, in fluoridation policies[4] and provision of services for priority groups.

What is accepted by the profession as good practice may not remain static but is subject to change. For instance, case law is an important source of law in the United Kingdom and can have a considerable impact on professional standards. The management of impacted wisdom teeth illustrates how changes in clinical practice can come about as a result. In the 1980s a number of court cases concerned residual numbness following the extraction of wisdom teeth.[11,12] The result of the debate within the profession is that dentists now recognise the importance of warning people about the possibility of numbness and fewer symptom-free wisdom teeth are extracted.

The National Institute for Clinical Excellence has now issued guidance for the removal of wisdom teeth.[13] This demonstrates that patients have the right to be told about significant risks that are known to be associated with a clinical procedure and the responsibilities that clinicians have to give patients that information before they consent to undergo treatment.

Ethical principles in healthcare

Historically the moral standards that govern clinical practice have centred on the importance of doing good (beneficence) and not harming others (non-maleficence). However, in recent years there have been two further important additions. Beauchamp and Childress, in *Principles of Biomedical Ethics* first published in 1979,[14] included the hitherto neglected principles of autonomy and justice in their formulation of bioethical principles. Their work therefore established four principles which are now widely accepted in the contemporary discourse of medical ethics.

Autonomy concerns respect for a person's capacity to determine what happens to them; in healthcare, this concerns what happens to their own body. In practice, this means that a person has a right to information and choice before deciding whether to accept any kind of clinical intervention. If autonomy is to be respected it is the patient rather than the dentist who must decide how his/her dental care is managed. But patients are not in a position to make such decisions unless a dentist shares with them their professional knowledge about the treatments that are possible together with any advantages and disadvantages. People have a right to control what happens to them when they attend for dental care and they should be involved in making decisions. Ozar and Sokol, in their book *Dental Ethics at Chairside*,[15] describe different models of the dentist–patient relationship depending on whether decisions are patient led or dentist led. They reject these models in favour of an interactive model where both dentists and patients enter into an interactive negotiation which is based on informed consent.

Rights to autonomy may at times compromise a person's welfare.[16] For example, from the dentist's perspective there may be obvious advantages in saving a tooth whilst a patient opts to have the tooth extracted. Nevertheless once the dentist has explained the options so that the patient can understand any possible consequences the patient must choose freely for him/herself if his/her capacity to be self-determining is to be respected.

Principles of justice call for all patients to be treated without prejudice, whatever their gender, race or class. For example, patients should not be discriminated against because they are HIV positive. Justice also calls for resources to be fairly distributed, based on need rather than income or status. A person who is elderly, sick or disabled has as much right to dental care as a young and healthy person. Indeed, how well care is provided for the most vulnerable and needy in a society is itself a mark of that community's well-being.

Ethical standards have most often concentrated on the obligations that health professionals have in providing healthcare. But this situation is now changing with the emerging emphasis on patients' rights. Newer rights-based moral theories are sometimes contrasted with the more paternalistic utilitarian theories of the past.

For example, confidentiality in providing healthcare is an ancient principle outlined in the Hippocratic Oath (300 BC)[17] where doctors affirm 'All that should not be spread abroad I will keep secret and never reveal'. A utilitarian moral argument says that patients will be much happier if they know that the dentist will not divulge to others any information about them or their dental treatment. Confidentiality may thus be seen as important to maintaining trust in the dental profession. On the other hand, a deontological rights-based argument says that people attending for healthcare have a right to privacy and confidentiality. It is unlikely that in the clinic either of these moral theories, or any other moral theory for that matter, operates in isolation and Beauchamp and Childress point out that in clinical practice different and even conflicting moral theories will often be operating together in a consensus.[14]

The importance of moral reciprocity in healthcare demonstrates that it is not the professional alone who has responsibilities. Patients too have obligations. For instance, a dentist has a responsibility to be available at the time arranged whilst the patient has the responsibility to attend for appointments. This principle of moral reciprocity is based on the golden rule of treating others as you would like to be treated. A dentist who keeps to time with appointments is more likely to have patients who attend on time whilst a dentist who consistently keeps patients waiting should not be too surprised if patients in turn do not always come at the agreed time.

In the same way dentists as well as patients have rights. Dentists should not, for example, be pressurised into providing unnecessary or inappropriate treatment that would go against their professional integrity. The dentist has the right to refuse to extract a sound tooth even though the patient adamantly requests that it is taken out.

The mutual recognition of rights and responsibilities in human interactions is an essential component of our common humanity. The obligations that people have to each other are informed by the generally accepted moral principles of the community. Doyal and Gough suggest that it is this capacity of human beings to recognise and exercise such reciprocity that makes social life possible.[18]

Rights and responsibilities therefore go hand in hand. A patient has a need to have a painful tooth treated whilst a dentist has the knowledge and skills to carry out that treatment in order to alleviate the pain. As these dual moral commitments are recognised in clinical care, more equal and healthier relationships are established between dentists and patients so that the provision of dental treatment becomes a joint activity and a greater partnership between those concerned.

The challenge of applying ethical principles in practice

It is one thing to articulate principles but it is not always so easy to honour rights and meet obligations. For instance, both doctors[19] and dentists[20] are finding it increasingly difficult to adhere to the stated ideals within the limits of available resources. This presents a challenge in wealthy western societies and even more so in the developing world. There are important debates about the relative value of public health measures and individual health-care as a way of managing disease. Dentistry is an example where public health measures have had an appreciable impact in reducing the levels of disease. This is not an either/or situation but rather both approaches have a place, but to neglect either one is to fail in professional obligations to recognise the rights to high standards of health and healthcare that individuals and populations have.

Although rights and responsibilities are of central importance for dental ethics and good professional practice, they have often lacked clarification in both regulatory mechanisms and dental education. Guidelines have been limited and patients have often invested an unquestioning trust in dentists. Ethics and law have not been systematically taught in dental schools. The teaching and learning of professional standards have been considered to be part of some informal hidden curriculum which remains assumed rather than being made explicit. But the situation is changing.

New educational guidelines from the General Dental Council[21] place a much greater emphasis on the need to include these subjects throughout the dental curriculum. Core topics that should be included have been agreed by teachers in British dental schools.[22] An understanding of rights and responsibilities, the importance of truthfulness, trust and good communication in clinical relationships, the importance of informed consent and confidentiality, the special responsibilities to those who are vulnerable or immature, professional duties of dentists, resource allocation and business ethics and dental research are topics identified as being essential for inclusion in the dental curriculum. They are each considered in more detail in later chapters.

Much has been written by theologians, philosophers and lawyers about ethical principles and legal theory but unless that theory is put into practice, it remains no more than theoretical idealism. In meeting professional obligations and respecting the rights of people in need, those who provide healthcare make moral theory a practical reality which informs human relationships. The discussion in this chapter can be summed up in the importance of courtesy and respect for human dignity. Whether it is a healthy woman, a young child or a sick elderly man who enters the dental clinic, the dentist has moral and legal obligations to do the best for that person. It is to be hoped that they will do so not through fear of censure but because they believe in the inherent worth of every human being and that is how they themselves would like to be cared for.

References and notes

1 Universal Declaration of Human Rights. United Nations 1948.
2 UN Convention on the Elimination of All Forms of Discrimination Against Women 1979.
3 UN Convention on the Rights of the Child 1989.
4 Montgomery J (1997) *Health Care Law.* Oxford University Press, Oxford.
5 Human Rights Act 1998.
6 Grubb A (1999) *Butterworth Medical Legal Reports.* Butterworths, Oxford.
7 Department of Health (1995) *The Patient's Charter and You.* DoH, London.
8 General Dental Council (1997) *Maintaining Standards: guidance to dentists on professional and personal conduct.* GDC, London.
9 General Dental Council (1997) *Duties of a Dentist.* GDC, London.
10 Hobdell M (1996) Health as a fundamental human right. *Br Dental J.* **180**(7): 267–70.
11 Heath v West Berkshire HA [1992] *3 Med LR* 57.
12 Christie v Somerset HA [1992] *3 Med LR* 75.
13 National Institute for Clinical Excellence (2000) *Guidance on the Removal of Wisdom Teeth.* NICE, London.
14 Beauchamp T and Childress J (1994) *Principles of Biomedical Ethics* (4e). Oxford University Press, Oxford.
15 Ozar D and Sokol D (1994) *Dental Ethics at Chairside.* Mosby, St Louis.
16 Rule J and Veatch R (1993) *Ethical Questions in Dentistry.* Quintessence, Chicago.
17 Mason J and McCall Smith K (1999) *Law and Medical Ethics* (5e). Butterworths, Oxford.

18 Doyal L and Gough I (1991) *A Theory of Human Need.* Macmillan, Basingstoke.
19 Richards P (1998) Professional self respect: rights and responsibilities in the new NHS. *BMJ.* **317**: 1146–8.
20 Grace M (1996) Editorial: rights and responsibilities. *Br Dental J.* **181**: 79.
21 General Dental Council (1997) *The First Five Years: the undergraduate dental curriculum.* GDC, London.
22 Bridgman A, Collier A, Cunningham J *et al.* (1999) Teaching and assessing ethics and law in the dental curriculum. *Br Dental J.* **187**(4): 217–19.

CHAPTER THREE

Professional duties of dentists

Amolak Singh

Dentists, especially general dental practitioners (GDPs), are often eager to attend postgraduate courses to learn new techniques to enable them to offer advanced treatments or cosmetic work, including implants. These areas can be most remunerative. However, it is often forgotten that this is the very type of work that attracts complaints that may lead to litigation. The safety of patients is paramount and should over-ride personal and professional loyalties.[1]

The Lord Chancellor, writing in the *Medical Law Review*,[2] has said that medical litigation is increasing and awards made by courts are often startlingly high. As dental technology advances and new materials come to the market, expectations rise and the consumer can become over-optimistic. Dentists or doctors cannot and should not guarantee success for any treatment undertaken. Patients have the right of self-determination, the right to a treatment plan with costs anticipated and the right to refuse any treatment. It is the duty of a dentist to respect these rights.

This chapter will cover the following topics.

- Professions and professionals: history and development
- Standards of care: duty of care to protect the life and health of patients
- The importance of continuing education
- Unethical and unsafe practice in dentistry: 'whistle blowing'
- Health and professional performance: risks, duties to disclose problems and sources of help
- Public expectations of dentistry; difficulties in dealing with uncertainty and conflict
- Ethical importance of good inter- and intraprofessional communication and teamwork

Professions and professionals: history and development

The history of dentistry dates back to almost the 5th century BC, with some forms of dental knowledge exhibited amongst the Phoenicians, Egyptians, Chinese, ancient Hebrews and Europeans.[3] In Europe those who practised dentistry in the 19th century were called 'surgeon-dentists'. They lacked any scientific knowledge and often inflicted harm on their patients.[3]

In England dental hospitals were established before dental schools. The first dental hospital opened its doors in 1858 in London. In 1860 the Royal College of Surgeons held the first examinations for the Licentiate in Dental Surgery, but it was not until 1878 that the first Dentists Act was passed authorising the General Medical Council to maintain a register of qualified dentists who could call themselves 'dental surgeons'. Unfortunately the Act did not prohibit those who were unqualified from practising dentistry, it only prevented them from calling themselves 'dental surgeons'. The untrained continued to practise without fear of prosecution.

In 1917 the government set up a committee to 'enquire into the extent and gravity of the evils of dental practice by persons not qualified under the 1878 Act'. On the basis of the report, the Dentists Act 1921 was passed. The stricter controls laid the foundations for the current system of regulation, with offenders liable to a £100 fine. The Act also prohibited corporate bodies from carrying on the business of dentistry unless certain conditions were met.

The 1921 Act gave the profession a measure of autonomy by setting up a Dental Board. Though under the control of the GMC, this was the forerunner of the General Dental Council. The 1921 Act permitted unqualified dentists to register if certain conditions were met, such as age over 23 years, being of good character and if dentistry was their principal means of livelihood in five of the seven preceding years.[3]

The 1956 Act granted the profession full self-government by establishing the General Dental Council, with powers to supervise dental education, maintain and publish the Dentist's Register and enforce standards of professional discipline. The 1956 Act was an amendment of the previous Acts. A consolidating Act was passed in 1957.

The European Dental Directives in 1978 required member states to adhere to common standards of training for primary and specialist qualifications and to permit migrant dentists with appropriate qualifications the freedom to work in the host state. Recognition of specialist qualifications was not implemented until 1998.

Then followed the Acts of 1983 and 1984. The Dentists Act of 1957 was improved and updated in 1983, including the establishment of the Health

Committee. The Act was consolidated in 1984, under which the profession still operates.

The Health Act 1999 received Royal Assent on 30 June 1999. Provisions of the Act enable the Secretary of State to make changes to the Dentists Act 1984 by Orders in Council. Hence primary legislation will no longer be required to amend the Dentists Act.[4]

Definition of a professional

A profession is an occupation requiring advanced education and involving intellectual skills, examples being medicine, dentistry, law, etc. It is a vocation or calling that involves some branch of learning or science.

A professional is a person doing something with great skill or one engaged in or worthy of the standards of a profession. The professional uses his or her knowledge by its practical application to the affairs of others, serving their interests or welfare.[5]

A successful professional is one who benefits mankind, has a fair degree of independence and is respected within his or her community.[5]

Standards of care: duty of care to protect the life and health of patients

In the ordinary law of negligence the conduct of the reasonable man is assessed. In medical or dental law the reasonable doctor or dentist is substituted for the reasonable man. The concept of duty is the key controlling feature of the modern law of negligence,[2] regardless of whether that duty arises in contract or tort. Reasonable conduct is not negligent,[6] unreasonable conduct can amount to negligence.

In Bolam v Friern Hospital Management Committee 1957,[7] Mr Justice McNair held that: 'The doctor is not guilty of negligence if he has acted in accordance with a practice accepted as proper by a responsible body of medical men skilled in that particular art'. The Bolam test was affirmed in the House of Lords in 1980.[8]

In Sidaway v Board of Governors of Bethlem Royal Hospital and Others 1985,[9] the standard of care was on the issue of what information should be given to a patient to obtain valid consent to treatment. It was held that the Bolam test applied. Lord Diplock said: 'In matters of diagnosis and the carrying out of treatment the court is not tempted to put itself in the surgeon's shoes; it has to rely on expert evidence'.

In Australia it is the courts, and not the profession, that determine the standard of care. In Canada Bolam was never accepted, as it would allow 'doctors to legislate themselves out of liability'.[10] In Reibl v Hughes in 1980,[11] the Supreme Court of Canada held that the doctor's duty was to provide information that a reasonable patient would wish to know.

Bolam was revisited in the UK in 1997 in Bolitho,[12] where the House of Lords upheld the principles of Bolam but reserved the right to intervene if medical opinion was not reasonable, not responsible or if it was illogical.

Duty to protect the life and health of patients

No treatment should be undertaken if it is going to harm the patient even if the patient specifically asks for that particular treatment. The patient's best interest should be the primary concern of the practitioner. The practitioner should say 'no' where appropriate.

The GDC maintains a serious view on the taking of medical history. History taking, both dental and medical, is a special form of the art of communication.[13] It informs dentists of risks that they may encounter and precautions that may be necessary. Practitioners are advised to make themselves familiar with the Dental Practitioners' Formulary and, if necessary, to communicate with the patient's medical practitioner.

Unnecessary exposure of patients to radiation must be avoided. Practitioners should be familiar with the Department of Health's publications *Radiation Protection in Dental Practice* and *Radiological Protection July 1988* and the Report by the Royal College of Radiologists and the National Radiation Protection Board 1994.

General anaesthesia is a procedure which is never without risk.[1] The GDC has published very precise guidelines on the use of general anaesthesia. Every surgeon has a responsibility to abolish pain during surgery but this should not be at the risk of endangering the patient's life.

The importance of continuing education

In its ethical guidance *Maintaining Standards*, the GDC states:

> In the interest of patients, a dentist has a duty to continue professional education whilst continuing to practise. A dentist who fails to maintain and update professional knowledge and skills and who, as a result, provides treatment which falls short of the standards which the public and the profession have a right to expect, may be liable to a charge of serious professional misconduct. (para. 1.3)

Each generation of professionals may on occasion accuse its predecessors of ignorance as standards of competence steadily rise.[14] Practitioners must exercise such care as accords with the standards of reasonably competent medical professionals *at the time*. They must keep themselves up to date and cannot 'obstinately and pig-headedly carry on with the same old technique if it has been proved to be contrary to what is really substantially the whole of informed medical opinion'.[14]

Lifelong learning: recertification for the dental profession

The GDC's Reaccreditation and Recertification scheme for the dental profession was launched at Dentistry 2000 in Birmingham. A preparatory scheme was introduced in October 2000. Dentists are expected to complete 250 hours of continuing professional development (CPD) activity over a five-year period. Not less than 75 hours must be 'verifiable' CPD while the remainder can be 'general' CPD. The scheme will become mandatory as soon as legislation permits.

The GDC's aim is to promote high standards to ensure the protection of the public through the profession's commitment to dental education. The concept of clinical governance was outlined in the government's White Paper, *A First Class Service: quality in the new NHS*. Recertification will ensure that all dentists update their knowledge and acquire new skills in order to benefit their patients and enhance the quality of their professional lives.

The scheme will operate in five-year cycles. At the end of five years dentists will have to declare the number of hours of verifiable and general CPD completed in the preceding five years. Registration will be conditional on completion of minimum hours specified in the scheme. The scheme will be widely publicised, monitored, scrutinised and, where necessary, dentists may be given additional time to comply. Non-compliance may lead to erasure. There will be a right of appeal to an independent review panel and a final right of appeal, perhaps to the Privy Council.

Unethical and unsafe practice in dentistry: whistle blowing

As a professional, a dentist has an obligation to put the patient's best interest before any self-interest. Para 3.1 of the GDC's ethical guidance says:

As a member of a caring profession, a dentist has a responsibility to put the interests of patients first. The professional relationship between dentist and patient relies on trust and the assumption that a dentist will act in the best interests of the patient. Abuses of this professional relationship may lead to a charge of serious professional misconduct.

It is unethical for a dentist to mislead NHS patients by saying that certain treatments are not available on the NHS when the statement is untrue. Once a patient has been accepted for NHS care then it becomes the responsibility of the dentist to provide all the treatment that is available on the NHS, which the patient is willing to undergo to secure his or her oral health.
  Some of the more common forms of unethical conduct are as follows.

- Providing composite restorations on posterior teeth without explaining the advantages and disadvantages of the filling material to patients, thus negating true consent.
- Instructing a dental technician to ask for denture work to be provided economically to meet NHS standards when the actual contract with the patient is for private work.
- Mixing of NHS and private work (which is permitted on NHS patients) without agreement and when genuinely the private treatment offered is not available on the NHS. Patients must not be misled.
- Over-prescribing treatment. All over-prescribing is deemed to be not only unethical but also to constitute an assault on the patient.
- Refusal to treat a patient solely on the grounds that the person has a bloodborne virus or any other transmissible disease or infection.
- Breaching patient confidentiality. A dentist so doing may be found guilty of serious professional misconduct.

Unsafe practice in dentistry occurs where there is:

- a lack of proper equipment
- poor record keeping and omitting to take an adequate medical history
- poor cross-infection control
- an incompetent practitioner or untrained staff, neither updating their professional skills
- undertaking techniques and forms of therapy which are unproven
- a dentist practising with a transmissible disease or a bloodborne virus
- impaired mental health due to drink or drugs or psychiatric illness
- non-compliance with health and safety issues
- undertaking sedation or general anaesthesia contrary to the GDC's ethical guidance.

It is not possible to list all forms of unethical conduct or unsafe practice in this chapter. Readers are referred to the GDC's ethical guidance *Maintaining Standards*, the BDA's Advice Sheet B1 *Ethics in Dentistry* and *Quality Systems for Dental Practice*.

Whistle blowing

Under-performing dentists bring the whole profession into disrepute. The GDC's ethical guidance in *Maintaining Standards* states that:

> A dentist must act to protect patients when there is a reason to believe that a colleague's conduct, performance or health threatens them. The safety of patients must come first at all times and should over-ride personal and professional loyalties.
>
> As soon as a dentist becomes aware of any situation which puts patients at risk, the matter should be discussed with senior colleagues or an appropriate professional body.

Under-performing dentists will not only get themselves into trouble sooner or later, but in so doing they will undermine public confidence in the whole profession, as did happen in Appleton v Garrett 1997 where a dentist was convicted for committing a battery on his patients.

The Public Interest Disclosure Act 1998 protects whistle blowers from being victimised. It was enacted to protect employees and is of only limited value in dentistry as most dentists are self-employed. In 1986 the Federation Dentaire Internationale (FDI) passed a resolution that discouraged whistle blowing. However, in today's climate of high expectations, and the direction from the GDC, whistle blowing has been made respectable in the interests of the public and the profession.

Where there is concern about another dentist it is best to discuss the matter with senior colleagues, defence organisations, professional associations and the dentist concerned. If there is no improvement the dentist should be warned that a complaint may be made to the health authority concerned or to the GDC. The aim should be, as a first step, to support and educate the dentist. At this stage confidentiality should be maintained.

> Networking is a powerful tool, with the advantage being that it is informal and flexible. Whistle blowing is an ethical issue determined by a mix of attitudes, values and culture. Although there will always be guidelines, it remains an unwritten code, self-regulated and voluntarily accepted.[15]

The GDC has approved a Performance Review Scheme which will be established when the necessary legislative framework is in place. The aim of the scheme will be to protect the public and to educate dentists whose professional performance is seriously deficient. An independent Professional Review Committee will be set up with the power to impose conditions on a dentist's registration and an erasure for non-compliance. There will be a right of appeal to the Privy Council or the High Court.

Health and professional performance: risks, duties to disclose problems and sources of help

Para. 4.2 of *Maintaining Standards* says:

> A dentist who is aware of being infected with a bloodborne virus or any other transmissible disease or infection which might jeopardise the well-being of patients, and who takes no action, is behaving unethically. The Council would take the same view if a dentist took no action when having reason to believe that such infection may be present.
>
> It is the responsibility of the dentist in either situation to obtain medical advice which may result in appropriate testing and, if a dentist is found to be infected, regular medical supervision. The medical advice may include the necessity to cease the practice of dentistry altogether, to exclude exposure-prone procedures or to modify practice in some other way.

Failure to observe the above guidance may lead to a charge of serious professional misconduct.

The current Health Service Guidelines HSG (93) 40 *Protecting Healthcare Workers and Patients from Hepatitis B* recommend that healthcare workers infected with hepatitis B who carry the e-antigen, a marker indicating high infectivity, should not perform exposure-prone procedures, where there is a risk that injury to the healthcare worker could result in their blood contaminating the patient's open tissues.

Health Circular 1998/226 supersedes the 1994 guidance on the management of AIDS/HIV-infected healthcare workers. It reflects the conclusions of an independent review commissioned by the Department of Health on the risk of HIV transmission from an infected healthcare worker to a patient. Dental students and all healthcare workers are advised to read the new guidance that can be obtained from the Department of Health, Communicable Diseases Branch, Wellington House, 133–155 Waterloo Road, London SE1 8UG.

Alcohol and drugs

Complaints of drunkenness or misuse of drugs can lead to a charge of serious professional misconduct or referral to the Health Committee of the GDC. A dentist should prescribe drugs only in connection with the provision of *bona fide* treatment.

The Sick Dentist scheme was established in 1986 to help dentists who needed medical attention. It also served to protect patients and the reputation of the profession. There are regional referees and a scheme co-ordinator. If a dentist feels that a colleague may be in need of help (and to protect him or her from a complaint to the GDC) he/she should telephone 0207 487 3119. This number is widely advertised in the dental press.

Public expectations of dentistry: difficulties in dealing with uncertainty and conflict. Ethical importance of good inter- and intraprofessional communication and teamwork

Public expectations of dentistry are well summed up in the GDC's booklet *The Duties of a Dentist.* The information in this booklet was designed for dental students and the public. The topic is covered elsewhere in this book (*see* Chapter 7).

Uncertainty and conflict

Uncertainty and conflict lead to mental arguments as to how to act in certain situations. The dentist has to choose between alternatives. The rules of confidentiality may present such a dilemma, but remember, like discretion, confidentiality can never be absolute. Justice Tobringer has said: 'The protective privilege ends where the public peril begins ....'.[16]

A request from the police to provide dental records of a patient may present ethical problems. There may be no problem if the records requested are only to identify a corpse. If patients intentionally want their whereabouts to be kept secret, they have every right to expect this and the dentist should not disclose addresses or any other information that may be used to trace them. Whenever faced with a dilemma a practitioner should carefully weigh the interest of society with that of the patient. If in doubt, advice should be sought from the defence body. A dentist, by law, has to help the police in a case where a crime has been committed. When a school telephones to ask if a child had a dental appointment, the dentist should co-operate if the child is very young, say under 10, but seek advice from the defence organisation if the child is older as maintaining confidentiality becomes important.

In one case a wife informed the practice that she was pregnant and was therefore exempt from NHS charges. She said that her husband would be attending later that day and he should not know about her pregnancy. After his treatment, at the reception, the husband offered to pay for his wife. The receptionist, not knowing what to do, went to the dentist for help. She told the husband that his wife did not owe anything. Where a patient specifically requests confidentiality, even if it is from a spouse, confidentiality must be strictly observed.

There may be instances where a wife may not want her husband to know that she wears dentures. She is entitled to her rights of privacy. Some patients may not wish even the postman to know who their dentist is or when they will be at the dentist (security reasons). That is why the GDC encourages dentists to send reminder cards in envelopes.

A dentist may wonder what to do when a young patient requests the extraction of a painful upper anterior tooth, refusing endodontic treatment advised by the dentist. If such a patient is fully competent (has the capacity to consent) and the dentist has explained the consequences of extraction and the patient still wishes an extraction, the approach may be to prescribe antibiotics for the infection and to recall the patient after a few days. Often, if pain has been relieved, patients may change their mind. Involve the parents if the youngster is below age 16.

If it is uncertain even after taking radiographs whether there is decay in a tooth, a practitioner may wish to keep the surface under observation. The suspicion must be recorded. Good and clear records must be maintained. Clinical opinions can differ but the dentist must always act in the patient's best interest.

When there is conflict, the principles of patient autonomy should be weighed against those of benefit to the patient. Professor Dworkin has argued that mild paternalism may be considered as a 'social insurance policy'.[17] Treatment must not be forced on any patient. The wishes of the patient should be respected and treatment refused if that may harm the patient.

Inter- and intraprofessional communication and teamwork

Communication remains a vital element in every relationship, be it between the GDC and the public, between the GDC and the profession or between the dentist and the patient.[18] This is equally true between the dentist and other members of the dental team: the hygienist, dental nurse, receptionist, dental technician and the practice manager. Good communication avoids misunderstandings in the dental team and adds to the efficiency of a practice. Sir Douglas Black, writing on the responsibilities of consultants, said:

> This wide field of communication is one in which all of us have still much to learn, sometimes sadly from our own mistakes. In the immediate present context, I would underline the importance of good communication in preventing complaints, and of bad communications in engendering them.[19]

The Royal Commission on the NHS reported that almost one third of inpatients did not consider they were given sufficient information about their treatment and care. Silence and half-truths under the guise of 'therapeutic privilege' will only add to vagueness and inconsistency, creating suspicion that undermines professional integrity.

Teamworking pervades all walks of life and is gradually becoming recognised as the concept for the future in general dental practice.[21] Dame Margaret Seward defines a dental team as: 'all members of the practice, clinical or hospital staff who are involved in the provision of oral healthcare to the patient'. The patient is an integral part of that team, with the dentist as team leader. Dame Margaret, a Director of Teamwork, has worked tirelessly to improve the recognition of individual members of the dental team. She says that: 'Fundamental to success is a realisation that decision making must be taken by the team and free discussions must be held amongst team members at regular intervals'.[20] Together Everyone Achieves More (TEAM). There are five volumes of Teamwork obtainable from: Teamwork Office, 19–21 Northumberland Road, Sheffield S10 2TZ.

References and notes

1   General Dental Council (1997) *Maintaining Standards*. GDC, London.
2   The Rt Hon Lord Irvine of Lairg (1999) The patient, the doctor, their lawyers and the judge: rights and duties. *Medical Law Rev.* 7: 3.
3   Bremner M (1954) *The Story of Dentistry* (3e).
4   General Dental Council (1999) *Briefing Paper for Law and Constitution Committee*. GDC, London.
5   Maynard K (1970) *Review of Dentistry: practice administration and ethics* (5e).
6   Kennedy I and Grubb A (2000) *Principles of Medical Law*. Oxford University Press, Oxford.
7   Bolam v Friern Hospital Management Committee [1957] *2 All ER* 118.

8 Whitehouse v Jordan [1981] per Lord Edmund Davies.
9 Sidaway v Board of Governors of Bethlem Royal Hospital [1985].
10 Anderson v Chasney [1949] Manitoba Court of Appeal.
11 Reibl v Hughes [1980] Supreme Court of Canada.
12 Bolitho v City and Hackney Health Authority [1998] *AC 232 (HL)*.
13 Swash M (ed) (2001) *Hutchinson's Clinical Methods*. WB Saunders, Philadelphia, PA.
14 Rogers WVH (1998) *Winfield and Jolowicz on Tort* (15e). Sweet and Maxwell, London.
15 Edgar G (2000) Whistle blowing: the big dilemma. *Independent Dentistry*.
16 Tarasoff v Regents of the University of California [1976].
17 Dworkin G (1972) Paternalism. *Monist*. **56**.
18 Seward M (1997) *General Dental Council Initiatives*. GDPA Report.
19 Black D (1985) *Consultant Responsibilities*. MPS Annual Report.
20 Seward M (1997) *Teamwork: sharing a learning experience*. GDPA Report.

CHAPTER FOUR

Resource allocation and business ethics

David E Gibbons

In civilised life, law floats in a sea of ethics.
(Earl Warren, *New York Times*, 1962)

Resources are limited. Therefore rationing of resources is necessary. Rationing is not new. Rationing is an ethical issue; in particular, it raises issues of justice and rights (particularly the right to health). Several approaches to rationing have been suggested and some appear to have been implemented without having ever been proposed as explicit rationing mechanisms. These approaches satisfy ethical principles to a greater or lesser extent. Dentists, as professionals, have a duty to consider the ethics of resource allocation at both the micro and macro levels. Such considerations are necessarily limited and highlight inadequacies in current resource allocation, but it is better to acknowledge these limitations and work within them than to fail to identify them in the first place.

Introduction

One of the major problems confronting any politician or healthcare worker concerns adequacy of resources. It has been suggested that even if the entirety of the gross national product of the United Kingdom was allocated to healthcare and health services it would still be insufficient. So, what is the most appropriate way of allocating resources? Dentists in their practice do it every day. Whether this is by conscious or subconscious decision is a point on which the reader might wish to reflect. The resource they are allocating and for which they have a stewardship responsibility is the most precious resource they have: themselves and their time. How they use their time and in what form of healthcare provision they work, what group of patients they serve and what type of treatments they undertake are all a result of how they have decided to allocate their resources. This also identifies the other side of the coin, which is those who will not receive treatment as a result of their decision. Similarly decisions made at a national level by central government concerning, first of all, how much money should be allocated, for example to health services relative to defence or education, and then how much for dental services within the healthcare budget, require consideration of what cannot be afforded as a result and the likely impact that that will have on the population.

Such matters of allocation against finite resources are covered by the ethical principle of justice, in this case distributive justice. When a society's structures for distributing resources are ethically sound we might describe such a society as just. Aristotle many centuries ago observed that where justice is considered appropriate, in general it has to do with treating like cases alike and different cases differently in proportion to their relative similarities and differences. How, then, should these similarities and differences be determined and, as a result, how should society's resources be distributed?

How much dental care ought to be available in a just society and to whom? Should it be solely dependent on birthright or social class or ability to pay?

Several different approaches have been proposed.

Equality or equity

Were everyone's needs the same, then a sound case in a just society for distribution could be that everyone should receive the same amount of resource. But, of course, needs assessment in healthcare identifies differences. What point would there be in providing resources to individuals who have no need of it whilst at the same time denying extra resource to those who have need? Could equality then be considered as equal access to care or, developing it further, equal access for needed care. Each of these could be further discussed in terms of criteria. What, for instance, do we mean by equal access to care? Does this just concern itself with geographical distribution and take no account of the different known barriers to receipt of care and differing needs of patients, let alone differing capabilities of practitioners? Similarly, for equal access to needed care, how is this to be interpreted in a just society?

The equitable distribution of resources would move this a stage closer to the Aristotelian proposal of each according to their needs. This, however, is not as straightforward as it might at first appear. How are these needs to be determined and by whom? There are those in society who feel they have a need for a perfectly aligned, 'white' dentition whilst others' needs are for the removal of pain and sepsis; the difference, perhaps, between non-essential and basic oral healthcare. This begs further questions concerning 'basic for what' or 'essential for what'? Others would relate their criteria to function. Does society have any norms in this regard? If the definition of oral health proposed in the Department of Health Oral Health Strategy for England and Wales 1994 were used then 'needs' are capable of a very wide interpretation.

> Oral health is a standard of health of the oral and related tissues which enables an individual to eat, speak and socialise without active disease, discomfort or embarrassment and which contributes to general well-being.

Such a definition, however, was produced by a working group of the profession and might, in that regard, be considered to be the aspirations of the profession for the population rather than the other way round – society defining its own norms or a negotiation between the two.

Clearly, however defined, all needs cannot be met. There are many competing views of need. As a result explicit decisions and value judgements have to be made and priorities chosen about which needs are addressed.

Some of the suggestions made for setting priorities and determining who should receive services are:

- by contribution
- by effort
- through the free market.

Contribution

The underlying principle here is that resources are distributed in proportion to the value of a person's contribution to society. Thus if they invest, by whatever means, in society they should receive proportional returns on their investment by way of benefits. Thus, ethically, the relevant differences in allocation of resource to people are a reflection of their contribution. Where, then, does this leave those who have not yet contributed, such as children, or those unable to contribute through unemployment, illness or disability or those who have contributed and have now retired? How are the relative values of contributors to be measured and by whom? There is no standard value or benchmark nor does such an approach look after those unable to look after themselves, as it would destroy the contribution principle on which it is based. For a healthcare worker with a duty of care, such an approach would be difficult to accommodate.

Effort or merit

This approach suggests resources should be allocated according to how hard an individual works rather than the direct contribution. Thus the harder you work, the greater your return. But what if all the hard work is of no value to society or, worse still, is detrimental to society, such as in the case of a hard-working criminal? The effort or merit approach would require values to be ascribed to certain occupations and again takes no account of those unable to work or who are not working through no fault of their own.

This approach must again be considered to be unethical for a dental professional as it would permit one section of society to have all the resources whilst others have none.

Free market

The free market view holds that all social arrangements and distribution of resources are the product of voluntary exchanges within society in a free market. As a result a just distribution could be considered as whatever distribution occurs as a result of freely chosen exchanges, without reference to such things as relative need, contribution or effort. The over-riding principle here is a respect for an individual's freely chosen actions providing they do not impinge or violate someone else's freedom.

Applying this approach to dentistry suggests that care is only provided by the practitioner to those who are able to pay, to those with equal need or some other basis which could be considered as just and ethical.

Even within the NHS, where theoretically a distributive justice structure is in place for all, people's resources of time and money, etc. vary greatly and those with greatest need may have very limited or non-existent resources (the inverse care law). As a result many people's needs go unmet and any services received are very limited, whilst others are able to receive sophisticated, advanced care.

When reviewing the distribution of dental personnel in the UK it is clear that a mixture of the previous three approaches is, to a greater or lesser extent, in operation. Dental personnel in the main both reside and practise in the more affluent areas of the country where they share the value systems in place. Where individuals in the community, by dint of their contribution or effort to society, have acquired sufficient resources or influence to maintain a certain standard of living, they are able to access dentistry through free market exchanges. The resulting maldistribution exacerbates inequalities in oral health between the 'haves' and the 'have nots'. This poses a major ethical problem for both the individual practitioner and the profession's organised representatives. To accept the required redistribution and subsequent control of the profession to match the need of the population would be to undermine the autonomy of the professional to decide where to practise and on whom to practise. Thus an alternative NHS strategy of encouraging the profession, through incentives or new methods of payment, to move into areas of greatest need is being employed. Pulling in the opposite direction is the incentive to a practitioner to move into an insurance-based or private practice in which professional autonomy is thought to be maintained and the free market approach operates.

The ethical dilemma posed by these approaches can be summed up by a consideration of the question 'Is dentistry for dentists or for patients?'. In asking the question it is recognised that the almost universal answer is 'both'. However, the importance of the question lies in which of the two groups has primacy. If it is dentists, then it could be suggested that dentistry is no different from any other business and the commercial model predominates. If it is patients, then it could be incorporated within the professional model.

The commercial model

Dental care is like any other commodity bought by consumers and being a member of a profession is no different in principle from the activities undertaken by any other trader.

Thus the dentist has a product to sell and negotiates a treatment plan with a patient to their apparent satisfaction without coercion, cheating or defrauding. The patient enters the contract or agreement on the basis of *caveat emptor*, buyer beware, and not on the basis of informed consent. Patients thus are the means by which the practitioner gains rewards and dentists are guided by the interests which best serve that end. Treatment decisions are made according to the economic goals of the practice, maximising profit.

When a situation arises in which the patient's and the practitioner's interests cannot both be served then there is the potential for conflict and no room for resolution. Potentially this places economic considerations above patient welfare. Where, then, is the dentist's duty of care?

A problem practitioners face, when constantly bombarded with new materials and techniques each claiming superiority over the other in terms of their effectiveness or their quality or their potential for profit, is whether they should recommend less than the best, the best or the optimum? Is this where the business maxim of quality being 'fitness for purpose' enters the discussion? The ethical dilemmas posed by each individual patient are a constant source of soul searching.

Should this treatment be an extraction, with or without prosthetic replacement? If so, should a partial denture (acrylic or chrome?), a bridge (resin bonded or fixed with prepared abutments) or an implant be used? Or should endodontics and advanced restorative treatment be undertaken? In whose best interests are the decisions made? Has *informed* consent been obtained? Was the information on which that consent was based truly two-sided and without bias? Too frequently and for obvious reasons (a practitioner has to make a living and/or satisfy their employer in terms of their productivity), occasions arise when financial and other considerations over-ride what is necessarily the ideal treatment for a patient and a compromise has to be struck.

Provided practitioners are able to satisfy themselves, and others if necessary, that the duty of care is being met, that the decision is not motivated solely by financial reward, then they could consider that they are not solely operating in the commercial model of dentistry and are practising as professionals.

The professional model

The basis of the professional model is that dentistry is a moral practice and dentists therefore are concerned with using their expertise to advance the welfare of patients. Thus they are doing for patients, within the ethical code of the profession, what patients wish to have done. The primacy of the dentist's duty of care is paramount. Dentists place the interest of others above their own.

The ethical code of a profession is determined by representatives of the profession in association with lay representatives. For dentistry in the UK, this is the General Dental Council and these codes of practice are to be found in their publication *Maintaining Standards*. As such, a profession involves:

- important and exclusive expertise
- training, education and registration

- autonomy of judgement
- professional obligations and codes of conduct.

The major difference between these two models is that within the professional model, the patient's welfare should be considered supreme and that within the provider–patient interaction is the influence (through its guidelines and ethical codes of conduct) of an occupational regulator.

Responsibilities of practitioners

So far, the responsibilities of the dentist and dentistry with regard to equitable distribution of their own resources to patients in receipt of their care have been considered. The wider responsibilities of the profession to those who, for one reason or another, are either not availing themselves or are unable to avail themselves of that care have not been reviewed. For every patient being seen by a practitioner, there are several others who are unable to be seen. How has the priority decision been made that patient A will be seen and patient B will not? Is it based on the approaches mentioned earlier? Is it based on relative need? Is it just based on value judgements? Where does a practitioner's duty of care begin and end? What are a practitioner's responsibilities for the oral health of the local community?

If practitioners can ethically satisfy themselves that they have none, then on closure of their practice at the end of the day, do their obligations cease, except for their own registered patients? What price prevention? What is the role for health promotion? As a profession, dentists accept that prevention is the first choice but how often is it practised? How involved are practitioners in promoting prevention beyond the financially rewarding area of their own patients? Is this a professional responsibility? If it isn't then can they ethically justify the stance adopted by some of not providing periodontal therapy or implants for a smoker but continuing to provide routine conservative care for a habitual 'sweet snacker'? If it is acknowledged that lifestyle and environmental factors are closely associated with oral health, doesn't the dental profession, by virtue of its exclusive knowledge and expertise, have some responsibility for informing policy makers of these associations and thereby encouraging prevention? This could be through water fluoridation, milk fluoridation, school meals policies, smoking cessation in public places, etc. Although each of these has ethical considerations nonetheless the public bodies, whether at local authority or national government level, have a legitimate concern over the health of their constituent public. Currently many of these organisations have a vested interest in the maintenance of the status quo, for instance national government through taxes on tobacco and alcohol, local schools through additional revenue from sales of snacks, use of vending machines, etc.

Lifestyle factors are not the sole responsibility of the individual. Increased choice comes with increased affluence. Many in society, however, are deprived of the ability to make many of the lifestyle choices the profession might recommend for their oral health. It could therefore be construed as unethical for a professional to promote a sanction, e.g. withholding treatment, against an individual who apparently does not conform to a recommended way of behaving. The professional does not own another's health and therefore has no rights over it. The empowering of patients respects their autonomy and recognises the dentist's duty of care. It also recognises that the social context in which individuals live is an important influence on their behaviour. Social and cultural norms are different and each is probably entirely appropriate for that set of circumstances, at that particular time, for those particular people. The element of 'control' that any individual has over his or her behaviour will vary enormously. Thus the application of sanctions against a patient, or making an individual feel guilty about his or her inability to put into practice what is recommended, could cause harm and offend against the ethical principle of non-maleficence.

As a profession, dentists have rights and they have responsibilities. In exercising these, they face many ethical dilemmas, not the least of which must be the need to determine priorities when there are finite resources. How can a dentist best serve the public whilst at the same time serving themselves? This chapter has endeavoured to highlight some of the issues.

CHAPTER FIVE

The clinical relationship

Christopher Dean

Introduction

Over the last 30 years there have been significant changes in the ethical underpinnings of the relationship between dentist and patient. The purpose of this chapter is to convey, using a broad-brush approach, how the ethical landscape of the clinical relationship has altered. With an understanding of current theories both the student of dentistry and the established dental practitioner alike will not only be afforded some practical guidance in their working relationships with individual patients, but also be equipped to reflect more deeply on their professional practice and the ethical challenges that are to be faced.

Dental ethics is no longer simply to be found in a list of do's and don'ts with which dentists must comply. Of course, the codified professional obligations, such as the GDC's published guidance to dentists on professional and personal conduct,[1] still play a very significant role in a professional's working life and indeed, to breach such codes will have profound consequences for the dentist. However, because of changes in society, the evaluation of what constitutes ethical practice within the clinical relationship has ceased to be the prerogative of the dental profession. Rather, the constitution of dental ethics must be determined by reference to a coherent theory of the clinical relationship derived from, and subject to, an ongoing debate between the profession, academics, government and, crucially, the public. Because of this broad contributing base, a legitimate theory must take account of prevailing ethical mores and fit with an underpinning general ethical theory that is pertinent to human relationships both inside and outside the clinical setting.

Power within the clinical relationship

For the clinical relationship theory to be valid it must address one of the central problems of the relationship, namely the power imbalance which exists between the dentist and the patient. Power has been described by de Jouvenal as the 'capacity to make others do what one wants them to do against their own desires and preferences and against their wills'[2] and within the clinical relationship the locus of power has traditionally been vested with the dentist. There are two types of reason why this may have been so: those that are not specific to the clinical relationship and those that arise out of the particular nature of the transactions that occur between dentist and patient.

Power imbalance

The potential causes of inequality of power distribution which are not specific to the clinical relationship include, amongst others, cultural, ethnic and racial differences, the socioeconomic group of the dentist *vis-à-vis* the patient, age, gender, sexuality and religious belief. Sources of inequality which are specific to the clinical relationship include the dentist's monopoly upon technical skill and knowledge and the dentist's unique position as the interpreter of information within the clinical relationship. Both factors are, of course, linked to the acquisition of a special status for the dentist within society external to the clinical relationship itself. Additionally, *inter alia*, the clinical setting itself, the violation of bodily integrity associated with penetration into the oral cavity during dental treatment, the vulnerable physical position of the patient and the debilitating nature of dental pain and treatment all tend to buttress the power imbalance.

The dentist as 'gatekeeper'

The dentist's traditional role as the 'gatekeeper' to dental care provides a formidable barrier to external interference as well as increasing the patient's dependence upon the dentist.[3] Some argue that protection for the patient can only be achieved by transparency regarding the balance of power between dentist and patient and open discussion of what counts as an appropriate use of power or, conversely, an abuse of power.[4] On that view a dialogue within the relationship becomes critical to allow for the appropriate use of power.

Trust and power

A direct consequence of the power imbalance within the relationship is that the patient is compelled to trust the dentist. In other words, trust arises as a mode of interaction because it cements the unbalanced clinical relationship. However, trust may be misplaced; of itself, it offers no protection. Bayles identifies six obligations which he argues that dentists owe to their patients if they are to be deserving of their patients' trust: honesty, candour, competence, diligence, loyalty and discretion.[5] There is little doubt that these duties put flesh on the bones of a clinical relationship, but there are questions about what makes these particular obligations special.

Autonomy

Protection for the patient may be derived from the principle of respect for persons. Central to such a principle is the concept of a patient's right to self-determination or autonomy. Autonomy is derived from the Greek 'self' and 'law' and understands the moral imperative as the agent's own freely and rationally adopted moral policy. The idea of an autonomous person involves more than just the capacity to act on particular desires or choices but rather suggests a more general capacity to be self-determining and therefore in control of one's own life. Autonomy is the moral principle that supports one's freedom to think, judge and act independently without undue influence.[6]

Power imbalance and autonomy

The principle that an individual has the right to hold and act on personal values and beliefs is just as valid in the clinical relationship as it is in all human relationships. Protection for the patient may be achieved by selecting a theory that affords a pivotal role of respect for persons. Such a theory will then redress the power imbalance by imposing Bayles' correlative duties on the dentist. So the answer to the question of why such duties may be regarded as special is that they help to ensure that the patient is able to act autonomously within the clinical relationship.

Truthfulness

The duty upon a dentist to tell the truth is critical in the clinical relationship for to fail in this respect is to engage in a type of manipulation or subversion which undermines the patient's personhood and may have a corrosive effect on trust. However, truthfulness is more than just the passing on of accurate information. It is expressed in an attitude towards the patient by the dentist that seeks to create open and mutually respectful communication. Of course, the case for truthfulness is not absolute and the ethics of withholding information is explored later. There are situations where truthfulness may not be appropriate, but these must be regarded as exceptional. Examples include the possibility of deceiving young children, those with mental impairment and others with a significantly diminished capacity for rational deliberation and choice. But even when a dentist is justified in deceiving such persons, their capacity or potential for rational deliberation must be considered.

So, we have determined that respect for autonomy is important within the clinical relationship. It is therefore necessary to examine how the principle is invoked within different ethical theories, in order to determine which is appropriate to drive the patient–dentist relationship.

Consequentialism

In healthcare the traditionally dominant group of ethical theories was consequentialism. This group of theories, of which utilitarianism is the most well-known example, maintains that the results or consequences of actions (or of rules for action) are what matter. This view has great resonance for dental practitioners who are taught technical skills and acquire experience which allow them to alleviate pain and suffering, restore function, improve aesthetics and so on. However, there are a number of significant problems that arise in using utilitarianism as the basis for a theory of the clinical relationship. In particular, by failing to safeguard respect for persons, utilitarianism ultimately fails to protect the patient from the power imbalance within the clinical relationship.

Deontology

An alternative group of ethical theories – the deontological theories, from the Greek word *deon* or duty – give explanations of the validity of moral obligations that do not reduce to calculation of consequences alone. The major religions offer such moral rules but perhaps the most significant non-religious deontological moral theory is that of Kant. According to

O'Neill, the formulation of Kant's work that has had the greatest cultural impact is the categorical imperative that demands that we treat 'humanity in your own person or in the person of any other never simply as a means but always at the same time as an end'.[7] By giving autonomy primacy, Kantian ethical theory successfully redresses the power imbalance in the clinical relationship. However, upon reflection it is also clear that an unfettered exercise of patient autonomy, generating correlative duties upon the dentist in the clinical relationship, could, *reductio ad absurdum*, lead the dentist into conflict with both professional and legal codes. Accordingly, although a Kantian ethical theory would provide the total protection that was sought for the patient against the inequality of the relationship, nevertheless most sources agree that dentists do have at the least *prima facie* obligations to avoid harmful acts and engage in welfare-enhancing acts and Kant has no central place for these principles.

A hierarchy of moral principles

In its application to dental practice, the clinical relationship theory should offer some practical assistance to the practitioner in resolving the ethical dilemmas that arise within dental practice. Ozar and Sokol have suggested that conflict between principles be resolved by the adoption of a hierarchy of values.[8] A helpful route to a supporting ethical theory for a hierarchy of values may be to revisit the proposition that such a theory is to be derived from a dialogue within society. Such a dialogue, albeit hypothetical, is envisaged within the social contract tradition. In this approach, a negotiation occurs between persons in a set of circumstances engineered to eliminate inequalities; circumstances described by Rawls as his 'original position'.[9] The purpose of this thought-experiment dialogue is to determine which moral principles would be chosen by the contractors and how they would be weighted in a just society. This approach is most valuable in the clinical relationship with its associated power imbalance. Diggs is illuminating when he describes contractarian morality as requiring that we 'join others in acting in ways that each, together with others, can reasonably and freely subscribe to as a common moral standard'.[10]

Resolving conflicts in practice

Society has accorded the dental profession the privilege and responsibility of providing dental care. It is arguable that social contract theory would recognise the value of this special position and that the contractors would conclude that the primary obligation of the dentist is to avoid compromising two of Ozar and Sokol's values: the patient's general and oral health. This may be achieved by placing the duty to avoid a harmful outcome as a consequence of a dental intervention (a narrow variation of the duty of non-maleficence) at the pinnacle of a hierarchy of moral principles. Precise drafting in this context would be important in order to avoid the absurdity where such an obligation would prevent a dentist from causing pain in order to resolve a dental problem, e.g. local anaesthetic before placing a restoration.[11] After non-maleficence would be ranked the right of respect for persons, generating, as has been discussed, a correlative duty to respect a patient's autonomy as the next most important principle, thereby addressing the power imbalance in the relationship. Then the principle of beneficence would follow, ranked below both non-maleficence and autonomy. This would ensure that there was a positive duty upon the dentist to promote general and oral health but that this duty could only be acted upon in so far as the patient allowed.

The patient as 'gatekeeper'

Using this ranking of principles, in a sense it is the patient who becomes the 'gatekeeper' to dental services, not the dentist. This ranking order ensures that the patient's value systems and beliefs drive the treatment agenda, while at the same time ensuring that society's role for the dental profession is not compromised by the extreme libertarian position of forcing the dentist to comply with all autonomous requests.

The interactive dentist and patient

Having considered the underlying ethical theory of the clinical relationship, Ozar's work in this area is particularly helpful in a consideration of the best operational model for the relationship.[12] He describes an interactive model which stresses a process of information exchange and negotiation between dentist and patient as various decisions are encountered. As described by Ozar, the interactive model recognises the unique and irreplaceable contributions that both dentist and patient bring to the clinical relationship.

The importance of communication

The key to successful implementation of the interactive model depends upon the development of a range of effective communication skills by the dentist, in order to facilitate the process of information transfer from patient to dentist and vice versa. It should be remembered that if the patient is to be protected from the impact of the power imbalance in the clinical relationship, then true transparency over the power distribution in the relationship has to be achieved. This necessitates that the dialogue between patient and dentist should include information exchange regarding the impact of issues that on the face of it fall outside the clinical ambit. Examples of these have been identified above and include information about, *inter alia*, cultural, ethnic, racial and religious value systems and expectations,

The patient's right to have his or her autonomy respected is valueless unless the model adopted for the clinical relationship demands that the dentist initiates and facilitates full exchange of information between patient and dentist and supports full articulation of patient choices. The interactive model complements the moral principles articulated by the social contract theory, resolving the power imbalance in the relationship by allowing the patient to retain control over decisions that involve personal moral values or lifestyle preferences, whilst recognising the dentist's superior technical knowledge.

The personal qualities of the dentist

But what of the personal qualities of the dentist? Do these have any moral importance? MacIntyre believes that the character of the moral agent is paramount.[13] Virtue-based ethicists view such qualities as integrity, conscience and good character as central excellences of the clinical relationship rather than simply providing a gloss on the dentist's adherence to moral principles.[14]

It is self-evident that certain qualities are desirable in a dentist but are they sufficient? Will the possession of such qualities ensure that the patient is protected within the relationship? Smith and Newton suggest that for the clinical relationship to grow, it must involve dialogue, with the healthcare worker and patient exchanging information in a regular and explicit way. However it is arguable that the existence of a 'conversation'[15] in a virtue-based clinical relationship, while it involves the patient, is reliant upon the dentist to provide protection for the patient's own interests. It is submitted that much more effective protection for the patient is obtained by the recognition of a right of respect for personhood and its expression through an interactive relationship.

Withholding information from patients

The practical application of the theory of the clinical relationship may be illuminated by considering the ethical boundaries of the clinical discretion to withhold information. There are three major ethical arguments that are used to support the withholding of information by dentists.[16]

The first argument is that the dentist's obligations of beneficence and non-maleficence over-ride any requirement to inform the patient. Those who adhere to this view believe that if the patient is given full information about a serious condition, then this may, if distressing, undermine patient morale, reduce the placebo effect and impair the patient's recovery.

The second argument in favour of withholding information has two limbs: namely that the dentist can never be certain of diagnosis or prognosis and therefore to give what can only ever be partial information is to mislead; and further, even if the dentist was certain of all the information about a condition, the patient would be unable to understand it.

The final empirical argument is simply that patients do not wish to be given information about their condition when it is severe, particularly if life-threatening.

Arguments against withholding information

The unilateral withholding of information by a dentist from a patient is an exercise in paternalism – a denial of the right to autonomy for, as outlined above, the exercise of autonomy is meaningless without adequate information about the patient's condition being given, in order to allow rational deliberation. Even from an extreme utilitarian viewpoint which might be thought to support such a position, there is still an argument in favour of informing patients, for patients' welfare can be expected to be increased by dentists dealing frankly and honestly with their patients.

Patient-centred approach

If social contract theory is to be preferred, notwithstanding the existence of a right to be told the truth as a facet of respect for persons, information may still be withheld by the dentist if to do so would prevent a harmful outcome, remembering the ranking of principles. On the face of it, this seems to offer less protection to the patient than utilitarianism. However, there arises the need to consider who is the appropriate person to make a determination regarding the likelihood of such harm arising. It is submitted that there is no logical support for the proposition that the dentist should always make the decision over whether or not a patient would be harmed by being given information. In most circumstances the only person equipped to make such a determination is the patient and this presents the dentist with a practical, not a moral problem.

What is good communication?

If the patient is to exercise autonomous choice and make the determination of whether or not information should be withheld for him or herself, then in order to facilitate this process the dentist must master a range of communication skills. In this context it is worth repeating Gillon's warning that communication with patients should not be an 'indiscriminate, casual, curt or unsupportive truth telling to all patients'.[6] Rather, the dentist should learn the art of sensitive questioning, offer to answer any questions that the patient may have and ensure that adequate time is provided within the consultation for communication, precisely in line with Ozar's interactive model of the clinical relationship. In that fashion the patient controls the decision making within the relationship and is ensured full protection.

Effective communication

The second argument in favour of withholding information from patients fails, in a paraphrasing of Gillon's words, because here the ethical issue of withholding information revolves around the question of what it is right to do with such knowledge of the truth as a dentist believes himself or herself to possess.[6] The question of information consisting of probabilities only is irrelevant as such are the common currency of daily life, while the patient's inability to understand is relevant only in so far as it requires the dentist to become a more effective communicator.

The final argument in support of withholding information may be redrafted as follows: autonomous patients, when confronted by potentially life-threatening conditions, exercise their right to choose whether or not to be given information and tend to request that information is withheld by the dentist. It is an important argument because it recognises that it should be the patient who determines how much, if any, information is withheld. The important moral issue then becomes: what does the individual patient want in the particular circumstances? Again, this may only be determined by the employment of an interactive model for the relationship, with the precondition that the dentist is an effective communicator.

Conclusion

Ethical codes created by dentists to serve the interests of dentists have been superseded by an approach to dental ethics that is shaped by a dialogue between dentists and other interests. The consequence of the dialogue is the development of a theory of the clinical relationship which is solidly rooted in a deeper ethical theory and also provides assistance to the practitioner in resolving ethical conflicts in clinical dentistry. Such a theory of the clinical relationship meets the central objective of ensuring that patients are protected against inequality within the relationship between dentist and patient.

The responsible use of power by practitioners is enabled by the adoption of a pluralist approach, stressing the patient's right to have autonomy respected and the dentist's duty of truthfulness, ensuring that trust is deserved. The theory also meets society's requirement for a residual check upon the moral demands of unfettered autonomy, by retaining a primary duty upon the dental profession of non-maleficence.

The ethical importance of integrity, conscience and the good character of the dentist have been explored. Ozar's interactive model and the critical role that the dentist's communication skills play in ethical dental practice have been stressed. Indeed, the dentist's ability to communicate effectively with patients is so important from an ethical perspective that it is arguable that the explicit teaching of communication skills in the undergraduate dental curriculum should be accorded as much significance as the teaching of technical skills. A dental profession that continues to deliver a high standard of care *and* communicates effectively with its patients will be well equipped to deal with the challenges of dental practice in the 21st century.

References and notes

1   General Dental Council (1999) *Maintaining Standards: guidance to dentists on professional and personal conduct*. GDC, London.
2   de Jouvenal B (1957) *Sovereignty*. Chicago University Press, Chicago.

3   Turner B (1987) *Medical Power and Social Knowledge*. Sage Publications, London.
4   Brody H (1992) *The Healer's Power*. Yale University Press, New Haven.
5   Bayles M (1981) *Professional Ethics*. Wadsworth, Belmont, CA.
6   Gillon R (1992) *Philosophical Medical Ethics*. John Wiley, Chichester.
7   O'Neill O (1991) Kantian ethics. In: P Singer (ed) *A Companion to Ethics*. Blackwell, Oxford.
8   Ozar D and Sokol D (1994) *Dental Ethics at Chairside*. Mosby, St Louis.
9   Rawls J (1971) *A Theory of Justice*. Oxford University Press, Oxford.
10 Diggs BJ (1981) A contractarian view of respect for persons. *Am Philosoph Quart.* **18**: 104.
11 Rule JT and Veatch RM (1993) *Ethical Questions in Dentistry*. Quintessence, Chicago.
12 Ozar DT (1985) Three models of professionalism and professional obligation in dentistry. *JADA.* **110**: 173–7.
13 MacIntyre A (1981) *After Virtue*. University of Notre Dame Press, Notre Dame, IN.
14 Smith DG and Newton L (1984) The physician and patient: respect for mutuality. *Theor Med.* **5**: 43–60.
15 Katz J (1984) *The Silent World of Doctor and Patient*. Free Press, New York.
16 Bok S (1978) *Lying: moral choice in public and private life*. Harvester Press, Brighton.

CHAPTER SIX

Confidentiality

Andrew Collier

Being a dentist gives us many privileges. One of these is the right to ask patients questions of a confidential nature. Moreover, there is a right to expect replies and the right to refuse to carry out treatment if those replies are not forthcoming. However, this privilege also brings with it an obligation to maintain this information as confidential.

The expectation of confidentiality is central to a patient's trust in a dentist and the obligation to maintain confidence has been a vital part of the code of medical ethics laid down throughout history.

The Hippocratic Oath states:

> All that may come into my knowledge in the exercise of my profession or in daily commerce with men, which ought not to be spread abroad, I will keep secret and will never reveal.

This ancient oath has been modified by the Declaration of Geneva to read: 'I will respect the secrets which are confided in me, even after the patient has died'.[1]

The words may have changed but not the ethical requirement.

The General Dental Council

The General Dental Council (GDC) make a clear statement with regard to confidentiality.

> The dentist/patient relationship is founded on trust and a dentist should not disclose, to a third party, information about a patient acquired in a professional capacity without the permission of the patient. To do so may lead to a charge of serious professional misconduct. A dentist

should also be aware that the duty of confidentiality extends to other members of the dental team.

Where information is held on computer, a dentist should also have regard to the provisions of the Data Protection Act.

There may, however, be circumstances in which the public interest outweighs a dentist's duty of confidentiality and in which disclosure would be justified. A dentist in such a situation should consult a defence organisation or professional organisation or other appropriate advisor.

Communications with patients should not compromise patient confidentiality. In the interests of security and confidentiality, for example, it is advisable that all postal communications to patients are sent in sealed envelopes.[2]

This GDC code of conduct gives two messages: on the one hand, that confidentiality is usually absolute and extends to all members of the dental team. In addition, in whatever format information is held, the obligation remains the same. However, the GDC also acknowledges that in certain circumstances the public interest outweighs the dentist's duty of confidentiality and disclosure of information is justifiable.

Absolute confidentiality

Confidentiality will almost always be absolute. It is a key requirement of good clinical practice. Patients will not reveal information to clinicians if they fear that it may be transmitted to others. Indeed, confidentiality forms the cornerstone of trust in any professional relationship. The patient must also be protected from the distress and possible stigmatisation and discrimination that may be caused if their privacy were betrayed.

In addition, from a collective standpoint, patients may be more inclined to seek healthcare, or at least not ignore health problems, if they can be confident that their privacy will be maintained.

However, the first question that must be asked is 'what information is confidential?'.

Confidential information

What constitutes confidential information? Are there any circumstances where the release of information is acceptable? Is it reasonable to tell a wife, who rings to ask if her husband is having dental treatment at your surgery, that, yes, he is there or should she be informed that the information is confidential?

Should information be given to a schoolteacher who telephones to check on the whereabouts of a pupil at a certain time? Should information be supplied to the police if they enquire whether a person suspected of a crime was having treatment at the surgery at a material time? Should a wife be informed that her husband is HIV positive when she does not know and the husband specifically demands that she is not told?

It may be helpful to consider the situation from the patient's position. It is reasonable to ask how we would feel about our own information being known to others beyond ourselves and our dentist. This is hardly an objective standard but should give an operator pause for thought. Should others be treated differently from what we would choose for ourselves? Fortunately, it is not necessary to make a purely personal decision for each case. The law provides many general answers for what constitutes confidential information.

The legal duty of confidence

Several noted court cases[3] have established the legal duty of confidence and developed the principle that there are three elements required to establish a breach of that duty.

- Information must have the necessary quality of confidence.
- Information must be disclosed in circumstances implying an obligation of confidence (this may be an inference drawn from the circumstances).
- Unauthorised disclosure would cause harm to the confider.

A further case, X v Y,[4] established that the harm to the confider need not be actual physical or psychological damage. The disclosure itself, with the potential for harm to the patient in the future, would be sufficient to establish a breach of the duty of confidentiality.[5]

This makes matters clearer. Within the dental practice, information imparted by the patients in relation to their treatment must be regarded as confidential. The circumstances of the healthcare environment would most definitely imply an obligation of confidence and unauthorised disclosure of this information would be in breach of this obligation whether or not actual harm occurred to the patient.

In addition, the GDC makes clear that the obligation extends to other members of the practice team. Dentists have a legal responsibility for the acts and omissions of their staff. Good staff training in this area is therefore essential. It must be emphasised that they must never talk about patients either inside or outside the practice. Breaches of confidentiality by staff, who have been made fully aware of their duties, would then be a serious disciplinary matter.

Dentists must be clear about their own obligations. Is it possible to acknowledge that one member of a family was present in the surgery at a certain time on a certain day if asked by another member of that family? The dentist must remain very cautious at all times. We may not know the circumstances of the situation or the reason why a request was made to us. There may be very serious ulterior motives behind a seemingly innocent question.

The dilemma about what is confidential obviously requires an individual assessment of the facts. However, apart from the legal guidelines above it is helpful to remember that personal health information, obtained in the course of consultation and treatment, is both confidential and, for the purposes of confidentiality, indivisible. Therefore no part of the information should, in normal circumstances, be disclosed to any third party, including relatives, not concerned with the treatment of the patient without the permission of the patient,[6] nor can information be selectively disclosed.

Nonetheless, the decision to disclose information or not may be an awkward one. Patients may have been attending a dentist for many years. They may be regarded as friends. However, dentists are bound by the legal and ethical code of the profession. The answer to a question to which we may not reply does not have to be 'I cannot tell you' or 'I do not wish to tell you'. A better form of words would be 'I'm afraid the ethical and legal code of my profession prevents me from giving you an answer to that question'. The refusal does not then come from dentists as individuals. The law therefore provides general principles that can be applied to individual situations.

The legally incapable patient

Does the duty of confidentiality apply to all patients? Consider the child patient or the patient who is mentally disadvantaged. Does the duty of confidentiality extend to them?

In the case of the child patient, the law states that there must be a definite age before which a patient does not have consent over their body. In addition, this must include the power of decision over confidential records about them. However, it has also been recognised that in practical and logical terms, there cannot be a sudden moment, based on age, when a young person acquires the necessary judgement and maturity for that capacity to consent. The patient who has, in legal terms, no right of consent on the night before their 16th birthday does not change significantly, in mental status, on the following day. In legal terms, it has therefore been clearly established in the case of Gillick[7] that consent, and legal rights to confidentiality, depend not just on age but also on understanding. If, in the judgement of the clinician, the patient has sufficient understanding and possesses sufficient intelligence to be capable of making up his/her own mind, then he/she should be able to control the disclosure of his/her own health records.

In the case of the mentally disadvantaged patient the same general rule applies. If patients have, in the opinion of the clinician, a sufficient level of understanding then they also have the right to consent to or refuse treatment and therefore, by definition, also retain the right of control over disclosure of their own health records.

However, what about mentally disadvantaged patients who have no understanding or, in the opinion of their clinician, insufficient understanding to consent to control over their own health records? This situation was clarified in the case of F v West Berkshire HA.[8] This was a medical case concerned with the sterilisation of a 36-year-old woman who had a mental age of 5–6. The court declared that:

> ... a doctor can lawfully operate on, or give other treatment to, adult patients who are incapable, for one reason or another, of consenting to his doing so, provided that the operation or other treatment concerned is in the best interests of the patient.

This case concerned consent in grave medical circumstances but it does establish a clear direction for all clinicians, including dentists, with regard to patient autonomy and hence the rights to confidentiality.

Justified disclosure

Having described reasons why patient information must, and should, be regarded as confidential, are there any circumstances where the disclosure of patient information *may* be justified?

It must be remembered that information belongs to the patient, not to the dentist. Therefore the patient may permit disclosure of any personal information to a third party. Third parties would include:

- other healthcare professionals participating in the care of the patient
- insurance companies seeking information in relation to injury claims, for example
- solicitors acting for the patient or for others.

However, are there certain circumstances where disclosure without the patient's consent, or even their knowledge, would be justified?

Such circumstances would be extremely rare for dental records but they do exist. The rule must be that there is either an individual justification, based on the individual circumstances of the situation, or there is a legal justification or obligation. The following situations may permit disclosure without consent.

- Where there is a legal or statutory requirement; this can include:
  - certain infectious diseases[9] (of which HIV is not one)
  - serious injury or dangerous occurrences[10]
  - certain Acts of Parliament.[11]

- When ordered to do so by a court. This requires an order from the court, not just a request from a lawyer or court official.[12]
- Where in particular circumstances, on medical grounds, it is considered undesirable to seek the patient's consent then information regarding the patient's health *may* sometimes be given in confidence to a close relative. This would be an extremely rare occurrence in dentistry and respect for patient autonomy remains paramount. As shown in a fairly recent medical case,[13] the existence of 'blood ties' alone does not confer the right to the acquisition of confidential information.
- When, in rare cases, it is justified in the wider public interest. However, as stated in the case of X v Y, 'It is well settled that there is a distinction between what is interesting to the public and what is in the public interest. It does not follow that simply because information would be of interest to the public it is in the public interest to disclose it'.[4] In two other cases the following principle was added: 'The public interest defence justifies disclosure to the "proper authorities", not necessarily to the world at large'.[14]

It must also be noted that disclosure may be justified in the public interest even if it affects just one member of the public.[5]

- For the purpose of a medical research project approved by a recognised ethical committee. In most cases the use of any patient material is dependent upon full consent to its use. However, certain research projects, by their nature and methodology, require the patient not to know. These factors will be carefully weighed and justified by a recognised research ethics committee. The dentist must be satisfied as to the validity of the research project.

- Identification of missing and deceased persons. Often the only method of identification of human remains will be dental records. If the dentist is satisfied that the release of confidential records *per se* is justified then this can be done. It can also be justified in order to minimise the distress of relatives.

Many of these situations will seem remote from a dental surgery, but the principles should be borne in mind. For example, consider a patient who suffers an epileptic fit in the surgery and then asks the dentist to keep this information confidential. He tells you that, as he is a self-employed lorry driver, he could lose his livelihood if he loses his driving licence. Although you attempt to persuade the patient to seek further help from his GP, he refuses and leaves the surgery. What should you do? You may have to decide whether to notify the patient's GP or the Driver & Vehicle Licensing Authority.

The General Dental Council states: 'There may be circumstances in which the public interest outweighs a dentist's duty of confidentiality and in which disclosure would be justified'.[2]

The decision must be based on the circumstances. In this particular case the patient may never have another fit. On the other hand, if he does, at the wheel of his lorry, he may cause death or serious injury, not only to himself but also to others. Is it therefore justifiable *not* to release the information? Duty to our patient may be outweighed by duty to society and other individuals.[15] This type of decision can be very difficult to make but the GDC ethical code of conduct does give guidance, as does the guidance from the British Dental Association.[6] Each situation, where there is any doubt, should also be discussed with a dental defence organisation before any action is taken. In the majority of cases an instantaneous decision is neither necessary nor justified. Time taken for reflection is usually time well spent.

Situations where there is a clear legal compulsion to release information, for example a court order, present no dilemma. The rule of law is absolute. However, other circumstances are less clearcut. It may be advisable in each situation to consider three questions.

- *Who needs to know?* This can present problems. The identity of the enquirer may be difficult to verify. Telephone requests for information should be treated with suspicion unless the person is well known. Meeting a relative or carer for the first time may require further verification of their status. Once again, an instantaneous decision could be unwise and delaying the decision to obtain more information may well be appropriate.

- *Why do they need to know?* The central question is: 'Can the release of the information be of benefit to the patient or conversely to the public at large, depending on the circumstances?'. If the answer is 'no' then release of information is not justified.
- *What grounds can justify the release of such information?* This third question really follows closely on the second. The clinician must make a decision that, although correct, may be very unpopular. Time for reflection is advisable and advice can be sought but the final decision and final responsibility rest with the clinician. He or she must be convinced that the decision is justified and if necessary, be prepared to defend that decision in court or in front of the GDC.

One final point to be considered when releasing information, with or without the patient's consent, is which part of the patient record or which item of information *needs* to be disclosed. If the whole record is released then more information than could be justified may be being given.

In conclusion, patient autonomy is paramount. However, in a small minority of cases it may be justified to give information. In these circumstances, the duty of confidentiality to patients can be breached.

Patient access to their records: the law

However, not only must confidentiality of patient records be maintained, there is also a requirement to maintain and keep secure patient records for their own access.

The right of access of the patient to their records has been evolving since legislation in 1970, superseded in 1981,[16] required the disclosure of medical records before a trial. This was to save time and prevent weak cases coming to court, which they would not do if both sides knew what the facts were beforehand. From this legal requirement there began a groundswell of public demand for access to, and the ability to correct, their own records. This has progressed as follows.

Data Protection Act 1984

This Act applied to any personal information held on computer record. A dentist needed to register with the Data Protection Registrar and comply with a series of data protection principles. In addition, patients had a right of access to their computerised records. The provisions of this Act have been maintained and enhanced by the Data Protection Act 1998 (see below).

Access to Medical Reports Act 1988

Patients acquired the right of access to reports made for insurance or employment purposes by a doctor or dentist.

Access to Health Records Act 1990

Patients received the right of access to their manual records made after 1 November 1991, subject to certain exceptions and exemptions, and also the right to request that an entry be corrected.

Data Protection Act 1998

This legislation extends the rights of patients regarding the 'processing' of information about them. It extends their control to prevent information obtained, by any healthcare professional, being used without their consent and requires that they are 'to be informed by any data controller whether personal data of which that individual is the data subject are being processed by or on behalf of that data controller'.

Patients therefore have a statutory right to examine, and an increasing right to control, their medical and dental records. There are very few legal exceptions to this right and it is almost impossible to think of any which would apply to dentistry.

Conclusion

In conclusion, the need to maintain confidentiality of any information given to us in our professional capacity is of paramount consideration. Patients have the ethical and legal right to expect this. Their trust in the maintenance of confidence is central to the success of the professional relationship with them. Confidentiality may be breached only with the patient's consent or if there is an overwhelming public interest in disclosure, either prescribed by law or based on our honest beliefs.

References and notes

1 Mason J and McCall Smith K (1999) *Law and Medical Ethics* (5e). Butterworths, London.

2 General Dental Council (1999) *Maintaining Standards*. GDC, London.

3 Hunter v Mann [1974] *QB* 767; Goddard v Nationwide Building Society [1986] *3 All ER* 264; A-G v Guardian Newspapers (no. 2) [1988] *3 All ER* 545.

4 X v Y [1988] *2 All ER* 648.

5 Jones MA (1990) Medical confidentiality and public interest. *Professional Negligence.* **17**.

6 British Dental Association (1995) *Ethics in Dentistry*. BDA, London.

7 Gillick v West Norfolk and Wisbech Area Health Authority [1985] *3 WLR* 83.

8 F v West Berkshire Health Authority [1989] *2 All ER* 545, HL.

9 Public Health (Infectious Diseases) Regulations 1988.

10 Reporting of Injuries, Diseases and Dangerous Occurrences Regulations 1995.

11 Prevention of Terrorism Acts 1974–89; Road Traffic Act 1988.

12 Administration of Justice Act 1970, ss 31 and 32 and the Administration of Justice (Scotland) Act 1972, s 1.

13 Re S (Hospital Orders: Court's Jurisdiction) [1995] *3 All ER* 290.

14 W v Edgell [1989] *1 All ER* 1089, 1104; A-G v Guardian Newspapers (No. 2) [1988] *3 All ER* 545, 659.

15 Brazier M (1992) *Medicine, Patients and the Law*. Penguin, Harmondsworth.

16 Administration of Justice Act 1970, ss 32–5 and Supreme Court Act 1981, s 33.

CHAPTER SEVEN

Consent to treatment

David Corless-Smith

Consent has both a moral and legal role to play and underlies the whole of medical practice.[1]

Introduction

It is axiomatic that the consent of a patient should be obtained before a dental examination or treatment is carried out. Few would argue that a dentist should be able to compel a patient to accept treatment, however beneficial to the patient. As a leading commentator has put it:

> no one, as far as I know, suggests that the millions of adults who stay away from dentists out of childish fear and to the detriment of their dental, and sometimes, their general health should be rounded up and marched to the nearest dental surgery for forcible treatment.[2]

However, that said, in dental practices up and down the country: 'Untold numbers of invasive, elective surgical procedures are routinely carried out without any apparent consent being either sought or given'.[3] Like many apparently self-evident assertions, when examined closely, the proposition that dental treatment should not be administered without the patient's consent becomes a little less straightforward.

Definition of consent to treatment

What is meant by consent in the context of consent to treatment? It is difficult to succinctly define the concept of consent to medical and dental treatment.[4] It is clearly more than simple agreement to treatment. Lord Diplock, in a leading case on consent to medical treatment described consent as 'a *state of mind* personal to the patient whereby he agrees to the violation of his bodily integrity'.[5] A basic, though far from complete, definition of the concept of consent to treatment is the voluntary submission to treatment following an understanding of the nature, purpose and consequences of that and alternative treatments.[6]

From this definition we can identify the three essential characteristics of consent to treatment, namely competence, voluntariness and knowledge. 'Competence' means that the patient has sufficient ability to understand the nature of the treatment and the consequences of undergoing or alternatively refusing the treatment. 'Voluntariness' means that the patient has freely agreed to submit to the treatment. 'Knowledge' means that sufficient comprehensible information is disclosed to the patient regarding the nature and consequences of the proposed and alternative treatments. These three elements are interdependent and for consent to be ethically and legally valid, all three elements must be present.[7]

In order to understand properly these constituent elements of consent to treatment, flesh must be added to this skeletal definition. However, the ethical foundation of the requirement to obtain a patient's consent to treatment must be considered.

The ethical basis of consent to treatment

The General Dental Council, in its ethical guidance to dentists in relation to consent,[8] states that 'a dentist must explain to the patient the treatment proposed, the risks involved and the alternative treatments and ensure that appropriate consent is obtained'. It is clear, then, that the concept of consent is held in high regard by the dental profession, such that a failure to obtain consent from the patient may amount to serious professional misconduct. But why should a dentist have to obtain the patient's consent before commencing treatment?[9] What are the ethical principles underpinning the concept of consent that justify its position as the 'cornerstone of moral dental practice'?[10]

There are two ethical principles which impact upon the concept of consent to medical or dental treatment: the patient's right to independent thought and decision making (principle of autonomy) and the dentist's duty to act in the best interests of the patient (principle of beneficence).

We must examine these ethical principles in some detail in order to understand the arguments for and against the necessity to obtain a patient's consent to dental treatment.

Autonomy

What is meant by autonomy and do patients have a right to have it respected? Autonomy[11] encompasses the notion that people have control over their own lives and are able to (and entitled to) make their own decisions as to their actions according to personal preferences and choices and without interference from others. The essence of autonomy is self-determination or, put another way, the unfettered ability to determine how one thinks or acts.[12] Thus an autonomous person can be said to have sovereignty over his or her own life.[13] In order to be autonomous, therefore, one has to be capable of thinking and acting freely without hindrance from others. Thus two conditions are essential in order to achieve autonomy: freedom from interference and capacity for independent decision making and action. But why is autonomy valued so highly? Why should a dentist respect the autonomy of the patient or, more generally, why should one respect the autonomy of other people? Harris describes 'respect for persons' as 'the starting point of morality'.[14]

Further, 'it is the starting point because it involves recognising that other people matter and so also that how they live their lives, and the quality of their lives, matters as well'. Thus Harris views respect for persons[15] as deriving from the intrinsic value of their life.[16]

There are a number of philosophical ethical theories which seek to justify the principle of autonomy. Perhaps the most important are consequentialism and deontology. The essence of consequentialism is that the rightness or wrongness of an act should be judged on whether its consequences produce more benefits than harms; that is, the outcome of the action determines whether it is ethically justified. This theory, of course, begs the definition of benefit and harm. There are many views on what counts as a good or bad consequence but they all consider that goodness, howsoever constituted, has intrinsic worth and that no further goal other than the achievement of a good outcome is necessary. Consequentialism thus conflates rightness and goodness. One form of consequentialism is utilitarianism whereby good consequences are measured in terms of happiness or pleasure and absence of pain.[17] Mill[18] justified the principle of autonomy (or principle of liberty, as he called it) on the grounds that its adoption leads to human happiness (which Mills considered possesses intrinsic worth and does not require its own independent justification).

The basic tenet of deontology[19] is that some actions are intrinsically right or wrong quite apart from their consequences and that a person only acts morally when acting under a duty to perform a moral action. Deontological theories differ in their derivative test of rightness. Probably the most influential deontological theory is that of Kant[20] who believed that rational human beings could identify moral duties according to his 'Categorical Imperative'. The essence of Kant's 'Categorical Imperative' is that people possess intrinsic moral worth and are entitled to equal consideration. There are three principles which comprise the test and all three must be satisfied if an act is to be considered moral. Paraphrased, the three parts are:

- act as if your action is to become law for everyone, yourself included, in the future
- treat other human beings as 'ends in themselves' and never as 'means'
- act as a member of a community where all the other members of that community are 'ends' just as you are.

All three principles involve recognising other people's autonomy. The first principle holds that no one has any more merit than anyone else and any moral action must be equally applicable to everyone.[21] The second principle emphasises mutual respect for each person's autonomy as to treat 'as an end' is to recognise that each person has his or her own purposes. The third principle stresses that each person in a community should respect the desires of others.[22]

Respect for autonomy is therefore, at its least, an acknowledgement of a person's right to make their own life decisions and hold their own views based on their personal values and beliefs without interference.[23] In the context of healthcare, autonomy translates to control over decision making that concerns one's bodily integrity, both physical and mental. It is the patient whose health is at issue and if a patient's autonomy is to be respected, ultimately it is the patient, not the doctor or dentist, who should take the decision as to what happens to his or her body. Thus respect for a person's autonomy demands that he or she should not be the subject of involuntary or unauthorised bodily interventions. It has been said that 'there can be no greater intrusion on a competent human being than to compel him to receive physical treatment that he does not want'.[24] If it is accepted that medical or dental treatment should not be compulsorily imposed, then the converse must also be true; that is, that the only therapy that would be argued for is that which is entered into freely, in the knowledge of the possible risks and benefits and with information as to alternatives where these exist.[25] Respect for a person's autonomy is a fundamental principle in dental ethics and is reflected in the necessity to obtain a voluntary and informed consent from the patient before any clinical intervention.

Beneficence

Traditional dental ethics holds that dentists should do whatever will benefit the patient. This is the principle of beneficence which is the moral obligation to act for the benefit of others.[26] But why should dentists be obligated to act in their patient's best interests? Is this just a definition of the job of a dentist – dentists care for the health (and oral health in particular) of their patients – or is there a duty to act in the best interests of patients beyond performing the job description? There is no doubt that this duty of beneficence towards patients is accorded a special status by the dental profession and this is reflected in the ethical guidance of the General Dental Council which exhorts that 'as a member of a caring profession … a dentist will act in the best interests of the patient'.[8] The principle of beneficence is readily justified as a moral obligation in consequentialist terms as the rightness of an action is defined as the promotion of benefits. Deontological theories, however, view beneficence as an imperfect obligation and distinguish between general and specific beneficence. A duty of specific beneficence is owed only to those with whom we have a special relationship. Outside such special relationships there is no duty of general beneficence and it is a matter of personal disposition as to whom we should help.[27] This notion of general beneficence is morally commendable but not obligatory. The dentist–patient relationship is considered to be such a special relationship which engenders a duty of specific beneficence on the basis of the dentist's assumption of responsibility for his patient.

A major problem with the application of the principle of beneficence in dental practice concerns how the patient's best interests are assessed. Does the patient's best interests relate to general health or specifically to oral health? And who should be the judge of the patient's best interests – the patient or the dentist? The dentist and patient may differ in their conception of what constitutes the patient's best dental interest. Dentists may legitimately differ in their consideration of what is technically the best treatment option for a patient. Even if such professional consensus is achieved, and assuming that the patient accepts the dentist's recommendation as to the technically optimal treatment option, the patient may take a different view of the best course of action to resolve a dental problem. A patient's life is only partly spent as a dental patient and a patient may reject an offered dental benefit in order to invest time and money to obtain another preferred non-dental benefit. Thus the notion of a patient's best dental interests encompasses a value judgement as well as a technical dental judgement. Where the patient's and dentist's views of what is in the patient's best interests differ there is a conflict between the dentist's obligation of beneficence towards his or her patient and the patient's right to have his or her autonomy respected. The relative priority of these moral principles creates dilemmas in dental ethics and nowhere is this more acute than in the context of consent to dental treatment.

Autonomy versus paternalism: the arguments for and against consent

Morality requires that not only should people's autonomy be respected but there should also be a contribution to their welfare. But should respect for an individual's autonomy hold a higher position in the moral hierarchy than the duty of beneficence towards another, especially when that beneficent act is imposed on another against his or her will?

Two extreme standpoints can be adopted as to the necessity to obtain a patient's consent prior to dental treatment. On the one hand, one can accept that the patient as an autonomous person is entitled to have complete control over decisions affecting his/her own body and any bodily intervention must be authorised. On the other hand, the rationale and primary goal of dentistry is to restore a person's well-being (or at least the well-being of their oral health) and dentists should be allowed to pursue this goal (which is of undoubted social utility) according to their perception of their patient's well-being without the necessity of obtaining the patient's specific authority to do so. The former view places a premium on respect for an individual's autonomy and the process of authorisation requires that all relevant facts that might influence his/her decision as to whether and in what manner his/her bodily integrity is to be interfered with should be disclosed. The latter view considers that the principle of beneficence should over-ride such respect for a patient's autonomy.

This deliberate over-riding of the patient's autonomy for the purposes of benefiting the patient is called paternalism. The moral justification of a paternalistic act is consequentialist in that it either protects patients from harming themselves or confers a benefit on the patient. However, this justification presupposes that the dentist rather than the patient is better placed to judge what constitutes a benefit or harm to the patient. In relation to treatment decisions the paternalistic dentist will assert that by virtue of his or her specialist dental knowledge and expertise acquired by training and practice, he or she is in a unique position to decide the most appropriate treatment plan for the patient. The argument goes that it would be impossible to educate the patient so that he or she could appreciate the technical intricacies of all the possible treatment options together with their risks and benefits and so the patient would not be capable of making a truly informed decision. Thus if the patient will not understand the information provided there is no point in providing it. Therefore treatment decisions can be, and ought to be, safely entrusted to the dentist.

However, we have already seen that dental treatment decisions properly involve an evaluative judgement of the patient's values and preferences as well as technical expertise. The dentist is not able to judge what will contribute to the patient's well-being (or even oral health well-being) by virtue of his or her technical expertise. Oral health is an evaluative rather than a purely technical concept and an informed patient is the final arbiter on how it is best achieved. The argument that there are practical difficulties in explaining the intricacies of dental procedures to patients can be overcome by better communication skills on the part of the dentist and does not justify non-disclosure of information to the patient.

Modern dental ethics has seen a paradigmatic shift from Hippocratic Oath-inspired paternalism to a human rights-based respect for autonomy. The priority now accorded to the ethical principle of respect for a person's autonomy within dental ethics generally is reflected in the recent renaissance of the concept of consent to treatment. Dental decision making was once considered the province of the dentist and the patient was rarely consulted regarding treatment choices. Paternalism prevailed. However, traditional dental ethics is increasingly coming under criticism. As Veatch stridently asserts: 'The Hippocratic oath is dead. No rational person would agree to it'.[28] The ethical obligation to obtain a patient's consent to dental treatment and the constituent elements of the concept of consent are now firmly rooted in the principle of respect for autonomy. As Gillian puts it:

> Even if one accepts a consequentialist position (according to which it is only the outcome of an action that matters morally speaking), paternalism is a suspect stance; and respect for people's autonomy seems to rule it out in general.[29]

We turn next to examine the individual elements of an ethically valid consent to dental treatment.

The elements of an ethically valid consent

As mentioned above, in order to achieve an ethically valid consent three requirements must be satisfied:

- the patient must be competent to consent to treatment
- the patient must have sufficient knowledge of the proposed treatment and its alternatives
- the patient must voluntarily agree to the treatment without coercion or undue influence.

Competence to consent[30]

This requirement might more accurately be seen as a precondition to giving valid consent rather than a condition of consent. Competence means the ability to perform a task. The criteria for determining whether someone is competent to perform a task depend on the nature of the task. In relation to competence to consent to dental treatment, the criterion is 'the degree to which the patient is able to understand and appreciate the information that is being conveyed during the consent process'.[10] Thus patients are competent to make a decision if they have the capacity to understand the information, to make a judgement about the information in accordance with their values and to communicate that decision.[31] There are four elements to this definition of decision-making competence: ability to understand information; stability of values; ability to make a judgement according to those values; and communication of the decision.

First, the ability to understand information provided by the dentist regarding treatment options requires cognitive and imaginative skills to process the information provided and appreciate a basic concept of the dental condition and its treatment options. The second requirement is awareness of and stability of personal life goals and values. Patients should have a conception of their values as regards their general well-being and oral health in particular. Also these values must be relatively stable over time. One's values change over a lifetime and especially during the emotional development of childhood and this is one reason why a child might be considered to be incompetent in relation to decision making. Third, competence requires that patients be able to reason and deliberate between the alternative treatment options by comparing the benefits and harms of the proposed treatment options in line with their goals and values and reach a decision as to their treatment of choice. Finally patients must be able to communicate their desired treatment option. Thus it will be seen that the criteria of a competent person and an autonomous person are very similar and that the concept of competence in decision making is akin to the concept of autonomy.

Patients will possess, in varying degrees, the abilities needed to satisfy the elements of decision-making capacity described above and in this respect decision-making competence is a continuum concept. However, decision-making competence is a threshold concept in that each individual patient will be competent or incompetent to make a particular decision. Further, competence should not be regarded as a 'global characteristic' such that a patient is competent to make all treatment decisions or none. But where does the threshold standard for determining decision-making competence lie? The standard varies with the complexity of the decision so that, for example, a patient may be capable of consenting to a simple amalgam restoration which requires a low standard of decision-making competence but incapable of consenting to complex orthognathic surgery. Some commentators have argued that the standard for decision-making capacity should vary in accordance with the level of risk of the procedure.[32] However, this combines the complexity of the decision and, the riskiness of the decision and, in the case of a simple low-risk procedure such as the extraction of an abscessed tooth, could lead to the conclusion that a patient has capacity to agree to the extraction but lacks capacity to refuse the extraction as non-treatment would carry a high risk of harm to the patient.

How is a dentist to assess whether a patient is competent to make a treatment decision? Various tests have been proposed for assessing competence.[33] The 'expressed preference' standard simply requires that the patient communicate a preference between treatment options. This standard does not enquire into the patient's reasoning process and the dentist could simply accept at face value any treatment decision made by the patient. The 'ability to understand' standard tests the patient's ability to understand the information provided about the treatment. The dentist explores the patient's appreciation of the risks and benefits of the treatment options (including no treatment). The 'actual understanding' standard equates competence with actual understanding and requires the dentist to educate patients and ensure that they have understood the risks and benefits of all treatment options. Finally the 'reasonable decision' standard judges patients' capacity according to whether their decision is deemed to be reasonable. Thus if the dentist considers that the treatment option chosen by the patient is not the best option for the patient then the patient's decision-making capacity is called into question.

It will be seen that the more stringent the standard of competence, the less respect is afforded to the patient's autonomy. Thus the concept of competence can be used as a device to over-ride the decisions of autonomous patients and treat them paternalistically. Indeed, in practice a patient's competence is only likely to be questioned if the patient chooses a course contrary to the dentist's recommendation, usually refusal of treatment. However, if a dentist could declare patients incompetent simply because they take a different view of where their best interests lie, the patient's right to self-determination would have little meaning. Therefore the appropriate standard for determining decision-making competence is ability to understand.

Knowledge

In order for patients to make an autonomous choice as to whether to submit to dental treatment, they must acquire the knowledge necessary to make an informed decision.[34] Without information, only guesses, not rational choices, are possible. So how much information must be disclosed to the patient regarding the proposed treatment? There are three possible standards of disclosure of information, determined by reference to, respectively, a reasonable person, professional practice and the actual patient. The 'reasonable person' standard requires information to be disclosed by reference to a hypothetical reasonable patient. What information would a reasonable patient want to know before making a treatment decision? At a minimum, the reasonable patient would want to know the nature and purpose of the proposed treatment, the material risks and benefits of the proposed treatment, any alternative treatment options together with their risks and benefits, the costs associated with each treatment option and the prognosis of the condition if left untreated. What risks should be disclosed? The more severe a potential harm of treatment and the higher the probability of occurrence of a harm, the more likely the harm would be considered relevant by patients in their risk–benefit analysis of the various treatment options. The dentist's fees would also enter into the risk–benefit equation as alternative treatment plans can vary in cost significantly.

The 'professional practice' standard sets the level of disclosure by the customary practice of the profession. This standard is likely to be less respectful of the patient's right to make an autonomous choice because the dentist will be acting out of a commitment to beneficence towards the patient and there will be a natural bias in favour of the proposed dental intervention which will accord with the dentist's conception of the patient's best interests and not necessarily with the patient's perception of his or her own best interests. Thus this standard allows paternalism to prevail over respect for autonomy. This is reflected in the concept of therapeutic privilege. Therapeutic privilege is the deliberate non-disclosure of information to a patient on the ground that such disclosure would be likely to cause the patient distress and suffering. In the context of decision making, it is usually the risks accompanying the dentist's recommended treatment plan that are not disclosed and the justification put forward is that the patient would place undue weight on such risks and irrationally decline to submit to the treatment option considered by the dentist to be in the patient's best interests. However, this plea ignores the fact that it is legitimate that the patient be influenced by anxiety in reaching a rational choice. Such anxiety is evidence that the disclosed information is relevant to the patient's values and life goals and therefore material to his or her deliberation. Without this information, patients are unable to exercise an autonomous choice. Thus the concept of therapeutic privilege is predicated on the paternalistic assumption that the dentist has particular insight into a patient's best interests which, as discussed above, is a dubious hypothesis.

The final standard of disclosure is the 'subjective' standard in which the adequacy of information is based on the needs of the individual patient rather than a hypothetical patient. This standard is the most respectful of the patient's autonomy and is the preferred ethical standard. How does the dentist know what information the individual patient would consider relevant to his or her treatment decision? This can be achieved by dialogue between dentist and patient so that the dentist discovers where the patient's values and goals lie in respect of his/her oral health well-being, enabling the dentist to tailor disclosure of information according to the patient's needs. It is argued by some that such a standard is too onerous, requiring that each patient is given a dental education. However, patients do not need to know technical minutiae in order to give an ethically valid consent. Rather, they simply want to know what harm and benefits may result from the alternative modes of treatment, including their severity and probability. It is not sufficient merely to provide the patient with all the relevant information; consent is only meaningful in terms of respecting a patient's right of self-determination if the information is actually understood. Many factors can interfere with a patient's comprehension, including extreme anxiety, fatigue and pain. The dentist should make an assessment of whether the patient has in fact understood the information.

Voluntariness

Lastly, for consent to be ethically valid it must have been given voluntarily as respect for autonomy requires that an individual's decisions are free from control by others. Control over a person should be distinguished from influence, which is resistible and therefore compatible with their autonomous decision making. Three categories of controlling behaviour have been described:[23] coercion, manipulation and persuasion.

Coercion can be defined as controlling another by the use of a credible and severe threat of harm or force such that the person is unable to resist acting to avoid the threat. Coercion always makes decision making non-autonomous and vitiates consent. Coercion is a rare feature of dental care but dentists may try to coerce a particular decision either because of what they perceive to be in the patient's best interests or to advance their own interests.

At the opposite end of the scale of control is persuasion, defined as influencing a person by use of an appeal to reason. Persuasion does not violate an individual's autonomy because he or she freely accepts as his or her own the viewpoint of the person persuading. A dentist can therefore attempt to influence a patient to accept a preferred treatment plan provided he or she is honest and objective in the reasons for the recommendation and is motivated by beneficence. Indeed, most patients will want to know which treatment the dentist thinks best.

In between these extremes of control lies manipulation which might be defined as influencing another through altering the choices available to that person or altering their perception of the choices by means other than coercion and persuasion. In the context of treatment decision making, manipulation may take the form of managing the information disclosed to patients in order to alter the treatment choices open to them or to distort their perception of those choices. Such manipulation is a deception and prevents patients making an autonomous choice because they are not acting on true information. Thus a dentist should not omit an acceptable treatment option or exaggerate or minimise the risks or benefits of any treatment option even if driven by beneficence. This would seem to rule out any use of therapeutic privilege to withhold information to manipulate patients into consenting to the dentist's recommended treatment.

Refusal of consent

Acceptance of the principle of respect for patient autonomy requires the dentist to respect a patient's choice if it is contrary to the dentist's recommended treatment. However, where the patient has refused a dental procedure that the dentist believes would be beneficial to the patient, it is incumbent on the dentist to be satisfied that the patient has evaluated properly the consequences of treatment and non-treatment and enquire into the reasons why the patient is refusing treatment. In this way any misunderstanding can be eliminated and the dentist can be assured that the patient has validly refused treatment. It should not be thought, however, that a patient's right of self-determination is a right to insist that the dentist provide whatever treatment the patient desires. Dentists are also entitled to respect for their autonomy and can refuse to provide the patient's preferred treatment if it is believed to be harmful.

The legal basis of consent

We next consider the law relating to consent to dental treatment and will examine whether the ethical basis of consent is reflected in the applicable legal framework.

So does the law of consent recognise the ethical principle of respect for a patient's autonomy or, put another way, does the law protect a patient's right to self-determination? The legal position in England is said to adopt the famous statement of Justice Cardozo:

> Every human being of adult years and sound mind has a right to determine what shall be done with his own body; and a surgeon who performs an operation without his patient's consent commits an assault [*sic*. battery] for which he is liable in damages.[35]

English law respects a person's autonomy and specifically protects a person's bodily integrity through the tort and crime of battery. Battery can be defined as any intentional non-consensual physical contact.[36] Thus any dental treatment which requires the dentist to touch the patient amounts to a battery and is unlawful unless done with the patient's consent (or another person authorised by law to consent on his or her behalf). This is so despite the fact that the treatment is beneficial to the patient and has been carried out with reasonable skill and there is no hostile intent on the part of the dentist.[37] Thus the requirement for consent means that the patient has a right to choose whether to accept or refuse dental treatment. The patient's consent licenses an otherwise unlawful act. Thus it has been said that the purpose of the requirement to obtain a patient's consent is to provide the doctor or dentist with a legal 'flak jacket'.[38]

We turn next to consider the elements of a legally valid consent to dental treatment.

Elements of a legally valid consent

The underlying jurisprudence of the law of consent follows the ethical analysis of consent adopted above; namely, for a consent to be legally valid it must be made by a person with capacity or competence to consent, it must be based on adequate information and it must be freely given without undue influence by others. Although the basic elements are the same as for an ethically valid consent, the precise requirements of each element differ.

Legal capacity

It is clear that there are individuals who are not capable, for whatever reason, of making decisions regarding their medical and dental treatment. Who should the law recognise as being capable of consenting to medical and dental treatment? There are two approaches that the law could adopt.

The law could pursue a status approach whereby an individual will be deemed legally capable (or incapable) to consent to treatment according to their membership of a particular category of patients which are either accorded or lack legal status to consent. So, for example, minors or mentally disordered patients might be deemed legally incapable to consent. A status approach to capacity is indiscriminate in that it does not look at whether an individual patient is capable of autonomous decision making.

The alternative approach to legal capacity adopts a functional approach in that the individual's actual ability to decide autonomously is tested. English law follows the functional approach. The patient must have sufficient mental capacity to understand what is involved in his or her medical or dental treatment. The legal test of capacity therefore tests the patient's facility or aptitude to understand rather than the actual understanding of the nature of the medical or dental procedures.[39] If the test of capacity required actual understanding on the part of the patient then a patient's capacity would depend in part on whether or not the dentist had disclosed sufficient treatment information. Thus patients could be rendered legally incapable of consenting simply because they receive an inadequate explanation from the dentist.

So what must a patient be able to understand in order to be assessed as legally capable to consent? Logically the level of understanding should relate to that information of which the law stipulates a patient must be aware in order to give a valid consent. However, the law distinguishes two levels of information that a patient should possess (see below). In order to avoid a battery claim, the dentist must inform a patient of the broad nature and purpose of the dental treatment. However, in order to avoid a negligence claim, the dentist must inform the patient of all viable treatment options and their risks and benefits, including those associated with no treatment. The law steers a middle course and requires that a patient be able to understand the nature and purpose of the treatment and the likely consequences of having or not having the treatment in question.[40] In the case of Re C (adult: refusal of medical treatment), the court developed a three-stage test[41] to assess a patient's capacity to understand which analyses the decision-making process thus. The patient must be able to:

1 comprehend and retain the relevant information
2 believe it and
3 weigh it in the balance so as to arrive at a choice.

This test of legal capacity is not concerned with the reasonableness or rationality of the reasoning process. Thus a competent adult patient has a right to consent to or refuse medical or dental treatment for reasons which are 'rational, irrational, unknown or even non-existent'.[42] As long as the patient has sufficient understanding of, and belief in, the consequences of undergoing or foregoing treatment and is capable of balancing the risks of accepting or refusing treatment against personal values and goals, the law will respect the decision as a competent one. However, if an ostensibly irrational decision is based on a misperception of reality then the patient might not be able to comprehend or believe the treatment information and therefore not satisfy the test of capacity.[43] Certain mental disorders can deprive a patient of the ability to make a true choice and such patients are therefore unable to satisfy the last stage of the legal capacity test. An example of relevance to dentistry is 'needle phobia' which compels a patient to panic and refuse a dental procedure. Such panic and fear could render a patient incompetent to consent to treatment.[44] Lastly, various external factors such as shock, fatigue, pain or medication might make a patient temporarily incapable of making a decision because the patient is unable to weigh the information and make a choice.[42]

Knowledge

In order to give a valid legal consent the patient must have an adequate knowledge of what is involved in the proposed procedure or in refusing it. This knowledge will usually be acquired from the dentist. How much information does the law require to be disclosed to a patient in order that consent be sufficiently informed?[34]

The law imposes two levels of duty of disclosure of information. The first and more fundamental level concerns that minimum level of information which must be disclosed to obtain a legally valid consent and a defence to a battery claim. The second more extensive duty relates to information in addition to the minimum level of information, which must be disclosed to obtain an 'informed' consent and avoid a claim in negligence. In the case of Chatterton v Gerson[44] patients' consent was held to be 'real' and legally valid if patients understand in broad terms the nature of the procedure they are agreeing to.

What is meant by the 'nature' of a procedure? The notion of the 'nature' of a procedure includes a factual description of the procedure to be carried out and its purpose and intended effect and also an understanding of the intrinsic quality of what is being done. In the case of Appleton v Garrett[45] a dentist carried out extensive unnecessary restorative work on healthy teeth for his own financial gain. The effect of deliberately concealing from the patients the fact that the treatment was harmful and unnecessary meant that they did not understand the basic character of what was being done and their consent to the treatment was invalidated. In other words the consent was secured by fraudulent misrepresentation of the basic nature of the act. But does an understanding of the 'nature' of a procedure include awareness of the risks inherent in a procedure? English law has decided that such matters are collateral rather than intrinsic features of a procedure and failure to disclose this information does not affect the validity of the patient's consent.[46] In some cases, who is carrying out the procedure may affect the nature and quality of what is being done. For example, if a patient is not aware that treatment is being carried out by a dental student, his or her consent may be invalidated if the treatment is in the nature of training rather than therapeutic care for the patient. However, in R v Richardson[47] the failure by a dentist to inform her patients that she had been struck off the dental register did not vitiate the patient's consent so as to render her criminally liable for battery. The patient's misunderstanding as to the defendant's qualification to practise did not affect the nature of the acts performed.

The law does, however, require a dentist to disclose information beyond the 'broad nature and purpose' of the procedure to encompass the risks and benefits of the proposed treatment and alternative treatment options, including the option of no treatment. In the case of Sidaway v Bethlem Royal Hospital Governors this duty of preoperative disclosure of information was held to be part of a doctor's overall duty of care towards his or her patient.[48]

The next question is how much information must a dentist disclose to a patient in order to avoid a negligence claim? The three possible standards of disclosure of information in relation to an ethically valid consent have already been considered. Which standard has the law chosen? In Sidaway[49] the House of Lords chose the professional practice standard. Thus the test of how much information a dentist should disclose to a patient is a rather circular one, namely that information which a reasonably prudent dentist would disclose.[50] This test can be criticised on a number of counts. First, empirically it is doubtful whether any such professional consensus in relation to information disclosure exists, even for relatively common dental procedures, so that the notion of a professional standard of disclosure is probably a fiction. Second, it presupposes that decisions regarding the appropriate level of information disclosure are solely a matter of clinical expertise. This ignores the distinction within dental decision making between the purely technical decision (which is the dentist's ambit of expertise) and the personal decision (which is uniquely that of the patient). Dentists have no special insight into their patients' values and their perception of their best dental interests and so cannot tailor their disclosure of information to that which the patient requires in order to make an informed decision according to their values. Instead dentists, acting in accordance with their perception of their patients' best interests, will want patients to accept their recommended treatment plan and will fashion their disclosure of information by failing to emphasise the risks involved in order to encourage acceptance by the patient.

This reluctance to deter a patient from agreeing to a particular therapy which is considered likely to effect a cure has been described as the 'therapeutic imperative' and is said to 'dictate much of medical practice'.[51] In adopting the professional standard of disclosure and accepting that explanations as to risks and alternatives are required only when dentists consider such information to be in the patient's best interests, the law has endorsed the notion of the 'therapeutic imperative'. However, in the recent case of Pearce v United Bristol Healthcare NHS Trust[52] the Court of Appeal appeared to resile from the professional standard and adopt the reasonable patient standard in requiring disclosure of significant risks associated a procedure which would affect the judgement of the reasonable patient.

Must the dentist make sure that the patient has understood what he or she has been told? Until recently the emphasis of the law had been on the duty of the doctor and dentist to disclose information to the patient and the question of the patient's understanding had almost totally been ignored. It is now clear that simply informing the patient is not enough; the dentist must give an explanation in terms which are reasonably comprehensible to the patient and take reasonable steps to ensure that the patient has understood the information.[53] However, this does not amount to a duty to ensure that the patient has in fact understood, which would be unduly onerous.

Voluntariness

The third element of a legally valid consent is that it must be freely given. Put another way, such consent must not be obtained by imposing unreasonable pressure on the patient. How far does the law recognise the controlling influences of others on a patient's freedom to consent to or refuse treatment? The leading case is Re T (adult: refusal of medical treatment) in which it was acknowledged that a patient's will may be overborne by more subtle influences than overt pressure. The test of voluntariness of a patient's consent is whether the patient's decision has been subjected to undue influence by others. The effect of the influence of others will depend on the patient's strength of will and their relationship with the person exerting influence. Clearly, then, coercion will render a consent invalid. The court accepted that persuasion, even strong persuasion, would not invalidate a consent. Thus dentists are entitled to persuade a patient to accept their recommended treatment option and to do so in strong terms if necessary, provided that they do not misrepresent the relative risks and benefits of the available options. However, the law will consider the power balance of the doctor–patient relationship especially in an institutional setting and will be alert to identify any coercive influences.[54]

Waiver of consent

Ethical considerations

Some patients may want only sufficient information to understand in limited terms their dental condition and are content to let the dentist treat their condition as the dentist sees fit. These patients do not want the responsibility of understanding their dental condition and being involved in treatment decision making. Such patients have a high level of trust in their dentist. In order to respect such a patient's autonomy it is important that the dentist carefully clarifies from the patient how much the patient understands about his/her condition and how much he/she wishes to understand. This will determine how much information the patient requires (and will be based on the patient's decision as to the degree of involvement in treatment decision making rather than the dentist's decision of what level of involvement from the patient is in the patient's best interests). In consulting patients' wishes in this way their autonomy is respected because patients have exercised their autonomous right to choose what is done to their body. The patient has exercised that right as much in declining information and involvement in decision making as in requiring information and involvement in decision making. Put another way, the patient has intentionally delegated his/her autonomy in decision making to the dentist.

The legal position

There is no obligation to disclose information where patients have indicated that they do not want to know but the dentist must be vigilant to ensure that the patient is willingly declining information.[55] However, it may be that the law does not permit patients to waive their right to be informed of the 'nature and purpose' of the procedure. Thus in law patients can waive their right to an 'informed' consent but may not be able to forego a 'valid' consent.[56]

Treatment without consent and proxy consent

Ethical considerations[57]

It has been argued that respect for a patient's autonomy requires a dentist to obtain a patient's consent before any dental treatment is carried out. However, some patients will lack the capacity to make autonomous treatment decisions for themselves: for example, young children by virtue of their underdeveloped cognitive skills and instability of life values, adults with cognitive deficits and the unconscious patient in an emergency situation. How should a dentist approach treatment of such patients? Strictly, respect for the patient's autonomy cannot be the guiding ethical principle as these patients are incapable of making autonomous choices. Although non-autonomous, these patients still warrant respect as persons and can be considered to have a right of self-determination which they are incompetent to exercise.

Treatment decisions on behalf of such patients must therefore be taken by surrogate decision makers and consent by a surrogate is called proxy consent. Even in an emergency, reasonable attempts should be made to obtain consent from an appropriate surrogate. The best surrogate decision maker is someone who knows the patient's values and preferences and will usually be a close relative of the patient. Surrogate decision makers can reach decisions on behalf of non-autonomous patients on one of two bases: a substituted judgement or a best interests standard. The former standard attempts to replicate the decision that the patient would have made had he or she been capable. This standard is only appropriate for incompetent adults who were previously competent. For children and adults who have never been competent the best interests standard is appropriate. Thus it will be seen that even in the case of incompetent patients the ethical principle of respect for autonomy prevails (as far as possible) over beneficence for the patient.

The legal position

We have seen that any physical contact without consent amounts in law to a battery. How, then, can dental treatment be given to patients who are legally incapable of consenting to treatment without the dentist incurring legal liability? We have identified three groups of patients who lack capacity to consent: young children; the mentally incapacitated; and the unconscious patient. The law treats each of these groups differently in relation to authorisation of medical and dental treatment.

Children have capacity to give a legally valid consent if they have attained sufficient intelligence to fully understand the nature of the proposed procedure and the consequences of either accepting or rejecting the recommended treatment.[58] If the child lacks the relevant capacity then a proxy consent on behalf of the child must be obtained.[59] Who can act as a proxy? The effect of the Children Act 1989 is that the rights and duties accorded by the law to a parent in respect of a child (which included the right to consent to medical treatment on behalf of the child) are now replaced by the concept of 'parental responsibility'.[60] Various people can have 'parental responsibility' under the Act. The court can also act as a proxy.[61] The proxy must exercise the right to consent on behalf of a child in the best interests of the child.

In the case of adults who are unable to give a legally valid consent, the law does not recognise anyone else as having authority to give or refuse a proxy consent. Nor is the court able to provide a proxy consent. Legal authority to treat an adult incompetent patient derives from the principle of necessity. In the case of Re F (mental patient: sterilisation)[62] the House of Lords decided that the legal mechanism for facilitating medical treatment for those adults who are unable to legally consent was to recognise that such treatment was necessary to preserve the health and well-being of the patient. Thus where a patient lacks legal capacity to consent, the necessity of the medical and dental treatment licenses what is otherwise an unlawful act. The test of necessity is judged by reference to whether the treatment is in the best interests of the patient, not by application of the substituted judgement test.[63]

Where a patient is temporarily incapacitated, for example an unconscious patient, the medical profession (and the law) has taken for granted that emergency treatment can be administered without consent in the patient's best interests. In the case of Re F the legal basis for the authorisation of emergency treatment was considered to be the principle of necessity. However, as the patient is only temporarily incapacitated a stricter test of necessity is imposed, namely that treatment is necessary to either save the life of the patient or prevent serious injury. Although it is good medical practice to seek the agreement of the patient's spouse or relative, such consent has no legal validity.

Lastly, we look at whether the law imposes any specification as to the form of a patient's consent.

Form of consent

What form can a patient's consent take? Strictly, consent is a state of mind whereby the patient agrees to submit to the proposed treatment. The law does not prescribe any requirements as to how a patient's consent is evidenced but two forms of consent are recognised: express and implied.

Consent is express where the patient explicitly agrees to the treatment. This may be orally or in writing. Consent forms are routinely used in hospitals when a patient undergoes a surgical procedure. The General Dental Council in its ethical guidance to dentists requires that written consent is obtained for the administration of general anaesthesia and sedation.[8] Consent is implied where it is reasonable to assume from the patient's conduct that he/she consents. The scope of implied consent should not be too widely construed. The fact that a patient enters the surgery and sits in the dental chair is implied consent to examination but nothing more.[64] Dentists carry out a wide range of procedures and the patient's open mouth is not to be regarded as *carte blanche* for dentists to carry out whatever treatment they wish.

Conclusion

The purpose of the ethical and legal requirement to obtain a patient's consent prior to undergoing dental treatment is to respect and protect patients' autonomy and right to self-determination and specifically their right to choose what is done to their body. A patient can only make an autonomous and informed choice about dental treatment following the provision of adequate intelligible information regarding the benefits and risks of the proposed and alternative treatments (and of foregoing treatment). Respect for an individual's autonomy demands that ultimately the treatment decision belongs to the patient, although the patient will be guided by the dentist's recommendation and be allowed to freely choose according to his/her conception of his/her best dental interests. Dental decision making involves both dental and personal decisions[65] and dentists are not justified in substituting their dental judgements for their patient's informed personal decisions. As McLean puts it:

> While it is accepted that the physician is the more competent to make the clinically appropriate decision, the patient remains the person who alone can take account of this clinical recommendation, evaluate it, and ultimately make a satisfactory personal decision'.[51]

So can it be said that the law promotes patient autonomy in medical decision making? There are many judicial utterances as to the fundamental importance of people's rights to determine what is done with their body and in particular to decide whether or not to consent to medical treatment.[66]

English law purports to respect patient autonomy by way of the tort and crime of battery which protects bodily integrity by prohibiting any non-consensual physical contact and the tort of negligence which protects the patient's right to choose whether to consent to dental treatment through the dentist's duty to disclose certain information regarding the treatment. The law differentiates between two types of consent according to the quality of information disclosure to the patient. The first type of legal consent can be considered to be a 'threshold' consent which requires only a knowledge of the basic 'nature' of the proposed procedure and is a defence to a battery claim. Clearly, then, the quality of consent which exonerates liability for battery does not even closely approach a vindication of respect for patient autonomy by the law. A patient can validly consent to a particular proce-dure with no knowledge of the risks involved in the proposed procedure and with no knowledge of potential alternative therapies. This level of consent is achieved without disclosing sufficient information to enable the patient to properly evaluate the recommended procedure against alternative options or in accordance with his or her values and goals regarding healthcare. As such, this type of legal consent does not satisfy the requirements of an ethically valid consent. It is a product of the judiciary's distaste for the use of the battery action against doctors or dentists who have failed to ade-quately inform their patients about their treatment which stems from the connotation of hostile intent that is traditionally associated with this claim.

The second type of legal consent is a more 'informed' consent which demands a knowledge of the risks and benefits of the proposed and alterna-tive procedures and is a defence to a negligence claim. Although this level of consent allows a patient to make a choice between available treatment options, it too fails to uphold respect for patient autonomy because it is the dentist who determines the level of information disclosure according to his or her conception of the patient's best interests and not the patient. Thus despite its rhetoric of proclaiming a patient's right to self-determination, the law of consent to dental treatment is predicated on the paternalistic principle of 'dentist knows best' and the patient's right of self-determination is barely protected. As Brazier puts it, 'the law of consent to treatment pays little more than lip service to patient autonomy'.[16]

Thus whilst an ethically valid consent is underpinned by the principle of respect for autonomy, a legally valid consent is presently firmly rooted in medical paternalism. However, there are signs that the law is becoming more sympathetic to the idea of autonomy with the recent emphasis on fuller disclosure and the need for the patient to understand the explanation of treatment given.[52] There are also signs that the paternalistic tradition of the dental profession is giving way to a new respect for patient rights. The General Dental Council in a document entitled *The Duties of a Dentist*, advise, *inter alia*, that a dentist must: 'have respect for a patient's dignity; listen to patients and respect their views and give patients information in a way which they can understand; and respect the rights of patients to be involved fully in decisions about their care'. These guidelines are all calls to respect a patient's autonomy and, although broadly expressed, approximate to the requirements of an ethically valid consent. If such guidance is heeded by the profession then the professional standard of information disclosure will come to equate with the ethical optimum of full disclosure and the gap between the ethical and legal requirements of a valid consent will disappear. Until then the dental profession is also paying lip service to respect for its patients.

As McLean laments: 'Patients should be in a position to avail themselves of professional services without inevitably rendering themselves vulnerable to denial of autonomy'.[51]

References and notes

1   McLean S and Maher G (1983) *Medicine, Morals and the Law.*
2   Brazier M (1992) *Medicine, Patients and the Law.* Penguin, Harmondsworth.
3   Matthews JBR (1999) *Risk Management in Dentistry.*
4   The *Oxford Concise English Dictionary* defines consent as '*v.i.* to concur, to assent, to agree, to yield, *v.t.* to agree to, n. acquiescence in feeling, thought or action, compliance, permission, agreement, concurrence'.
5   Sidaway v Bethlem Royal Hospital Governors [1985] *1 All ER* 643 at 658 (my emphasis).
6   See the definition of consent to treatment in *A Guide to Consent for Examination and Treatment* (1990) Department of Health, HC(90)22: 'The voluntary and continuing permission of the patient to receive a particular treatment. It must be based upon adequate knowledge of the purpose, nature and likely effects and risks of that treatment, including the likelihood of its success and any alternative to it'. See also the definition of informed consent in Gillon R (1992) *Philosophical Medical Ethics.* John Wiley, Chichester: '*a voluntary* uncoerced decision, made by a sufficiently *competent* or autonomous person, on the basis of *adequate information* and deliberation, to accept or reject some proposed course of action which will affect him/her' (my emphasis).
7   The ethical and legal threshold tests of sufficiency of each of the elements differ, however, as discussed later in the chapter.
8   General Dental Council (1999) *Maintaining Standards: guidance to dentists on professional and personal conduct.* GDC, London.
9   The General Dental Council's *Maintaining Standards*, in common with most professional codes of conduct, offers prescriptive guidance on standards of behaviour rather than critical ethical analysis.
10   See Hirsch A and Gert B (1982) Ethics in dental practice. *JADA.* **113**: 599 for an analysis of the role of consent in ethical dental practice.
11   The word autonomy derives from the Greek *autos* 'self' and *nomos* 'rule'.

12 The principles of autonomy and self-determination are synonymous.

13 See Beauchamp TL and McCullough LB (1984) *Medical Ethics*. Prentice Hall, Englewood Cliffs, NJ.

14 Harris J (1985) *The Value of Life: an introduction to medical ethics*. Routledge, London.

15 Harris[14] uses the term 'person' in a technical philosophical sense. He defines a 'person' as 'any being capable of valuing its own existence' (pp. 7–27). The concept of personhood is important in medical ethics because it defines to whom moral obligations are owed. There is much philosophical debate regarding the defining features of personhood. See further Gillon R (1985) *Philosophical Medical Ethics*. John Wiley, Chichester, pp. 41–53.

16 For further discussion of the concept of value of human life see Harris[14] and Glover J (1990) *Causing Death and Saving Lives*. Penguin Books, London.

17 Utilitarianism is also known as 'hedonistic consequentialism'.

18 Mill JS (1985) On liberty. In: G Himmelfarb (ed) *On Liberty*. Penguin, London.

19 The word deontology derives from the Greek word *deon* and means study of duty.

20 Kant I (1948) Groundwork of the metaphysic of morals. In: HJ Paton (ed) *The Moral Law*. Hutchinson University Library.

21 This principle is also known as the principle of universalisability and is equivalent to the golden rule of Christian ethics: 'do as you would be done by'.

22 For a readable introduction to Kantian ethics, see Seedhouse D (1998) *Ethics: the heart of health care*. John Wiley, Chichester, pp. 117–23.

23 See further Beauchamp TL and Childress JF (1994) *Principles of Biomedical Ethics*. Oxford University Press, Oxford. Chapter 3, 'Respect for Autonomy'.

24 Gostin LO (1982) Compulsory treatment in psychiatry: some reflections on self-determination, patient competency and professional expertise. *Poly Law Rev.* 86: 86.

25 McLean SA (1989) *A Patient's Right to Know: information disclosure, the doctor and the law*. Dartmouth.

26 This traditional duty to do good is accompanied by an obligation to do no harm (the principle of non-maleficence), i.e. dentists must also protect their patients from harm. Some argue that the principles of beneficence and non-maleficence are a single principle with the promotion of well-being and the avoidance of harm representing opposite ends of a continuum which includes the removal of harm and the prevention of harm. See further Beauchamp and Childress (1994), Chapters 4 and 5 and Rule JT and Veatch RM (1993) *Ethical Questions in Dentistry*. Quintessence, Chicago, pp. 53–6.

27 This limited range of application of the principle of beneficence is an argument for distinguishing the principles of beneficence and non-maleficence as the latter principle is of general application, i.e. it is a perfect duty.

28 Veatch RM (1981) *A Theory of Medical Ethics*. Basic Books, New York.

29 Gillian R (1985) Autonomy and consent. In: M Lockwood (ed) *Moral Dilemmas in Modern Medicine*.

30 See generally on decision-making competence: Hirsch and Gert[10] and Beauchamp and Childress.[23]

31 Ozar DT and Sokol DJ (2000) *Dental Ethics at Chairside* (2e). Georgetown University Press, Georgetown. *See also* Beauchamp and Childress.[23]

32 Brock DW and Buchanan AE (1989) *Deciding for Others: the ethics of surrogate decision-making*. Cambridge University Press, Cambridge.

33 Roth L, Meisel A and Lidz C (1977) Tests of competency to consent to treatment. *Am J Psychiatry*. **134**: 279.

34 The disclosure of information element of the concept of consent to treatment has been emphasised in medical law and ethics literature and has spawned its own doctrine of informed consent. This doctrine is considered further in Chapter 8.

35 Schloendorff v Society of New York Hospital (1914) *211 NY* 125 at 126.

36 The least touching of another's person ... is a battery; for the law cannot draw the line between different degrees of violence and therefore totally prohibits the first and lowest stage of it; every man's person is sacred and no other having a right to meddle with it, in any the slightest manner.' Blackstone (1830) *Commentaries, Book 3*.

37 Re F (mental patient: sterilisation) [1990] *2 AC* 1.

38 Re W (a minor) (medical treatment) [1992] *4 All ER* 627.

39 Gillick v West Norfolk and Wisbech AHA [1985] *3 All ER* 402.

40 Re C (adult: refusal of treatment) [1994] *1 WLR* 290; Re MB (medical treatment) [1997] *2 FLR* 426.

41 The three-stage test of legal capacity formulated in Re C was approved by the Court of Appeal in Re MB.

42 Re T (adult: refusal of treatment) [1992] *4 All ER* 649 per Lord Donaldson MR.

43 *See* Kennedy I and Grubb A (2000) Consent to treatment: the competent patient. In: I Kennedy and A Grubb (eds) *Principles of Medical Law*. Oxford University Press, Oxford, pp. 142–4; Kennedy I (1992) Consent to treatment: the capable person. In: C Dyer (ed) *Doctors, Patients and the Law*. Blackwell Science, Oxford, pp. 56–7; Kennedy I and Grubb A (1994) *Medical Law: text with materials*. Butterworths, London, pp. 137–48.

44 [1981] *QB* 432, 443 per Bristow J 'Once a patient is informed in broad terms of the nature of the procedure which is intended, and gives her consent, that consent is real'; approved by the Court of Appeal in Sidaway v Governors of Bethlem Royal Hospital [1984] *1 All ER* 1018.

45 [1997] *8 Med LR* 75.

46 Chatterton v Gerson; Sidaway v Bethlem. However, some commentators have argued that certain risks, if sufficiently serious and probable, ought to be viewed as a basic rather than collateral feature of a medical act and failure to disclose such features ought to incur liability in battery. See Sommerville M (1981) Structuring the issues in informed consent. 26 *McGill LJ* 740; Keng Feng T (1987) Failure of medical advice: trespass or negligence? 7 *LS* 149.

47 [1998] *43 BMLR* 21 (CA).

48 Sidaway dealt specifically with warnings of inherent risks of a procedure but subsequent cases have confirmed the duty to advise on the prospect of success of a procedure and of alternative therapies. *See* Gold v Haringey Health Authority [1988] *QB* 481 and Thake v Maurice [1986] *QB* 644.

49 As interpreted by the Court of Appeal in Gold v Haringey Health Authority.

50 This is the 'Bolam' test of liability which determines liability in all aspects of a dentist's duty of care. Thus a dentist is not liable in negligence if he has acted 'in accordance with a practice accepted as proper by a responsible body of medical [*sic.* dental] men skilled in the particular art'. *See* Bolam v Friern Hospital Management Committee [1957] *2 All ER* 118 and generally in Chapter 11.

51 McLean S (1989) *A Patient's Right to Know: information disclosure, the doctor and the law.* Dartmouth.

52 [1999] *PIQR* 53. This was achieved by synthesising the decisions in the cases of Sidaway (which applied the Bolam test to the duty to disclose information) and Bolitho (which reinterpreted the Bolam test). *See* Bolitho v City and Hackney HA [1998] *AC* 232 and Chapter 12 for discussion of modification of Bolam test by Bolitho.

53 Smith v Tunbridge Wells HA [1994] 5 *Med LR* 334.

54 Freeman v Home Office (No. 2) [1984] *1 All ER* 1036.

55 Sidaway per Sir John Donaldson MR.

56 Kennedy I and Grubb A (1994) *Medical Law: text with materials.* Butterworths, London.

57 The concept of proxy consent is considered in relation to children and mentally disabled adults in Chapters 9 and 10 respectively.

58 Such a child is said to be 'Gillick competent'.

59 The law also confers on a proxy a concurrent power to consent to treatment on behalf of a 'Gillick competent' child, thus denying a competent child the right to refuse consent.

60 Section 3(1).

61 Under the '*parens patriae*' jurisdiction under which the Crown as sovereign has a duty to protect its vulnerable subjects, including children.

62 [1990] *2 AC* 1.

63 Airedale NHS Trust v Bland [1993] *AC* 789.

64 Seear J and Walters L (1991) *Law and Ethics in Dentistry.* Wright, Bristol.

65 Segal H and Warner R (1979) Informed consent in dentistry. *JADA.* 99: 957.

66 Examples include: 'I start with the fundamental principle, now long established, that every person's body is inviolate ... the effect of this principle is that everybody is protected not only against injury but against any form of physical molestation ... Patients have a decisive role in the medical decision-making process. Their right of self-determination is recognised and protected by the law'; Re F (a mental patient: sterilisation) [1990] *2 AC* 1 per Lord Goff. 'An adult patient who suffers from no mental incapacity has an absolute right to choose whether to consent to medical treatment, to refuse it or to choose one rather another of the treatments being offered'; Re T (adult: refusal of treatment) [1992] *4 All ER* 649 per Lord Donaldson MR.

CHAPTER EIGHT

Informed consent

Andrew Bridgman

> At its core, it is respect for the patient as an individual, not as a defense against the possibility of later malpractice suit.
>
> (Jory Graham)

The phrase 'informed consent' appears frequently in the dental literature, but it is often used with considerable imprecision and consequently there is much misunderstanding of its meaning. First, it is often expressed as a legal requirement prior to the treatment of patients. On this understanding the provision of information may be seen as nothing more than a requirement to satisfy institutional or (perceived) legal rules. From this perspective the giving of information is simply that: *warning* the patient of risks inherent in the proposed treatment. Obtaining a patient's signature on a consent form to acknowledge this warning, or recording the same in the patient's notes, may be seen as nothing more than an elaborate ritual to protect against legal liability.

Second, the phrase itself is a misnomer, or at least misleading, implying perhaps that there is a difference between 'consent' and 'informed consent'. In actuality, for consent to be ethically or legally valid it must always be an 'informed' one. The difference, if this is a difference, lies in the cause of action upon which to base a claim. As demonstrated later, a claim for lack of consent lies in trespass (battery) and a claim for lack of 'informed consent' lies in negligence.

Third, it implies that the provision of information is simply to obtain the patient's agreement to go ahead with the proposed treatment. This is not so because the doctrine is broader than merely agreeing to treatment. The provision of information is a necessary ingredient in the patient's decision-making process. From this perspective, 'informed consent' is about enabling choices in recognition of a patient's right to self-determination. If, following the provision of information about proposed treatment, a patient chooses to go ahead then he or she will have given an 'informed consent'; conversely, if the choice made is to decline, he or she will have made an 'informed refusal'. Whatever the decision, it will have been his or her 'informed choice'.

This chapter proposes to clarify the meaning of the phrase 'informed consent', placing it in its proper ethical and legal contexts. It will do so through exploration of the dentist's obligations arising from the doctrine, from both moral and legal perspectives. In particular, it will examine the legal requirements and standards concerned with providing information and the tensions that exist between ethics and the law.

History

The doctrine of 'informed consent' has emerged comparatively recently in the philosophy of healthcare. The Hippocratic Oath, the fundamental moral code for the practice of medicine, makes no reference to the involvement of patients in the decision-making process. There was, of course, no need, perhaps for two reasons. The doctor was committed to 'follow a system or regimen which, according to my ability and judgement, I consider for the benefit of my patients'. The doctor knows best and thus there is no need to involve the patient when deciding the therapeutic regimen.

In addition, throughout the development of medicine and until recent times there was very often no choice in what treatment could be offered. This paternalistic approach to care, where doctors were able to rely on their own judgement for patient care, remained the predominant model for healthcare. Although there is evidence of consent seeking and information giving long before this time,[1] the concept of involving patients in the management of their illness through informed and shared decision making, the true doctrine of informed consent, was not an ethical issue until the latter half of the 20th century.

It has been considered that the catalyst behind this attitudinal shift was the Nuremberg trials at the end of World War II. The Nuremberg Code resulting from those trials suggested that the voluntary consent of the human research subject is absolutely essential and that consent should be based on sufficient knowledge and understanding. In the following years this approach extended to include medical treatment in general. However, it is likely that these changes owed more to societal influences outside medicine than to changes from within. Patients became more aware of the fact that choices could be made in many aspects of their life and more aware of their right to be involved in decisions which affected their lives; and that they could only participate in this process if they were 'informed'.

The concept of 'informed consent' is traditionally recognised as a 'transatlantic doctrine' that has its origins in the civil rights era in the America of the 1950s and 1960s. As usual, the law evolved to support such rights, the moral right to be involved in the decision process becoming upheld by placing a legal duty upon the medical profession to tell the patient of 'any facts which are necessary' to that process.

The moral perspective

In essence, then, the doctrine of 'informed consent' concerns itself with patient autonomy and the right to self-determination. Autonomy may be crudely defined as a person's ability to decide and act on the basis of rational thought and deliberation. It can hardly ever be described as pure because it is restricted by factors such as the law, society, the autonomy of others and personal circumstances (such as age and wealth). Professor John Harris describes four other, more specific, features or 'defects' that can further diminish a person's autonomy. Important in the context of this chapter are 'defects in the information available to the individual, upon which she bases her choices'.[2] Such 'defects' may arise, first, because the information is not provided either in part or in total or, second, because the person does not understand the information in the manner that it is given. The moral perspective of 'informed consent' clearly requires full disclosure and understanding in order to satisfy and uphold the principle of patient autonomy.

From this perspective patients are:

> entitled to receive sufficient information in a way that they can understand about the proposed treatments, the possible alternatives[3] and any substantial risk or risks which may be special in kind or special to the patient, so that they can make a balanced judgement.[4]

The legal perspective

'The ethical principle that each person has a right of self-determination finds its expression in law through the concept of consent.'[5] The common law has for centuries recognised the right of every individual to pass through life free from unwanted and unpermitted bodily intrusions.[6] The medical profession has been, for almost as long, no exception to this rule[1] and despite attempts by the court to limit liability,[7] the doctor or dentist who operates without the patient's consent will be *prima facie* liable for a battery (commonly called assault) in the tort of trespass to the person.

In law, for a consent to be valid, or real, it must be one that is given by a person who is competent to do so, given voluntarily and informed. The issue of competence is covered elsewhere in this book (p. 81). Whether or not consent is given voluntarily illustrates one other 'defect', identified by Harris,[2] that can diminish a person's autonomy: a defect in control; that is, the inability of the patient to act on the information. The law has given support to such a defect, for example, when the patient is on the trolley about to be wheeled into theatre,[8] or where there are external influences such as undue influence.[9]

This chapter is concerned with 'informed consent' and the question is therefore: how much information does the law require?

Nature and purpose

A series of cases, beginning in 1981, have clearly established the amount of information necessary for a patient's consent to be valid as an adequate defence to battery. Two cases in particular, Chatterton and Sidaway, make it clear where the law stands on this point. In both these cases the treatments for which the patients had consented carried certain known inherent risks. Unfortunately, those risks materialised and each was left in a worse condition. Mrs Chatterton and Mrs Sidaway argued that because those risks were not disclosed to them they were unable to make a proper choice and hence their consent was not real.

In Chatterton it was stated that: '... once the patient is informed in broad terms of the nature of the procedure which is intended, and gives her consent, that consent is real ...'.[10] This opinion was endorsed in the House of Lords in the case of Sidaway. It was accepted that Mrs Sidaway had given her consent to the operation because in signing the consent form she had declared that 'the nature and purpose of the operation had been explained to her'.[11]

It is clear that a patient's consent to surgery or treatment would be valid as a defence to battery even if he/she were not informed of any risks. Patients who agree to have their wisdom teeth removed will have given a valid consent to their removal if they are aware of the 'nature and purpose' of the operation, seemingly basic information.

Because of the recurring infection it would be wise to remove this lower left wisdom tooth. We will do it under local anaesthesia by making a small cut along the gum, and it will probably be necessary to take a bit of bone away so that we can lift the tooth out.

Without informing the patient of the risk of nerve damage, this is still a valid consent to an allegation of battery. Even if that risk materialises the patient will have no remedy in the tort of trespass for a battery.

Risks and alternatives

Agreeing to surgery with no knowledge of inherent risks is a substantial 'defect of information' which must severely diminish a patient's ability to make an autonomous choice. It would appear, then, that the ethical principle of a patient's right of self-determination is inadequately expressed through the concept of consent. However, this is not to say that this right is not supported at all by the law. In Chatterton it was stated that: 'the cause of action on which to base a claim for failure to go into risks and implications is negligence'. Thus the law strives to uphold the principle of self-determination and seeks to control 'defects of information' through the tort of negligence.

Duty of disclosure

In recognition of the patient's need for information the law has embodied the giving of advice within the duty of care owed to patients by a healthcare professional. Further, the giving of advice has been interpreted to include not only the risks involved in the proposed treatment but the options and risks of alternative treatments. Failing to satisfy that duty may expose the dentist to a claim in negligence. Negligence, and its complex rules, is fully discussed in Chapter 12, but in relation to the giving of advice the leading case is that of Sidaway.[11]

In 1974 Mrs Sidaway underwent an operation to relieve pain in her neck, shoulder and arm. The operation was intended to relieve pressure on the IVth cervical nerve by widening the vertebral foramina with 'dental burrs'. The operation carried a small risk of damage (2%) to the nerve roots and a smaller risk of damage (1%) to the spinal cord. Unfortunately for Mrs Sidaway the 1% risk of damage materialised and in consequence the operation left her severely disabled. Mrs Sidaway contended that the surgeon did not inform her of that risk and that in not doing so he had failed to fulfil his duty of care in respect of giving her appropriate advice.

In 1984 when the case came before the House of Lords it was established law that the appropriate standard of care in relation to diagnosis[12] and treatment[13] was determined by the 'Bolam test'. The question was whether such a test should apply to the duty of disclosure. Whilst standards of diagnosis and treatment were clearly matters for medical judgement, should the level of disclosure be similarly determined? It was held that:

> Whether non-disclosure in a particular case should be condemned as a breach of the doctor's duty of care is an issue to be decided primarily on the basis of expert medical evidence, applying the Bolam test.

The evidence before the court was that at the time of the operation, although some surgeons would have warned a patient of risk of damage to the spinal cord it was also accepted opinion not to have warned a patient of such a known risk. Mrs Sidaway failed in her action because a doctor 'is not negligent if he acts in accordance with a practice accepted at the time as proper by a responsible body of medical men ... merely because there is a body of opinion that takes a contrary view'.[14]

Standards of disclosure

Sidaway established a 'professional standard' for determining the amount of information to which a patient is entitled and such a position seems particularly unsupportive of the principle of patient autonomy. The level of disclosure is left to be decided by the profession and any redress for what may be a serious 'defect of information', such as that denied Mrs Sidaway, depends on professional opinion. Provisional opinion may be satisfactory to determine whether or not a dentist has arrived at a proper diagnosis or carried out appropriate or satisfactory treatment; these are matters that can be judged solely by the medical profession. In the context of decision making and disclosure of information, however, considerations other than clinical expertise or technical proficiencies are significant, considerations such as the patient's personal circumstances and wishes. This is no better illustrated than when elective surgery is being contemplated, as in Sidaway, where the operation to relieve pain carried a risk (measured at 1 in 100) of leaving Mrs Sidaway in a much worse condition. There can be no doubt that only the patient can make a balanced judgement between continued pain and the risks of surgery. For the profession to determine whether the patient need be told of those risks is far removed from any notion of patient autonomy and self-determination.

A better standard in support of self-determination would be the 'particular patient' standard, because it would recognise the individuality of each patient. Such a standard, however, would be difficult to satisfy as the patient may not know what information is required or may not be able to process the information believed to be necessary. It would also attach impossible obligations upon the doctors to assess each patient in order to determine what information would be relevant and enable him or her to make a decision. The alternative to the 'professional standard' is, then, the 'reasonable or prudent patient standard'. It is, perhaps, second best in comparison to the 'particular patient' test but pragmatically it is the best achievable. This is the standard that gave rise to the doctrine of 'informed consent' in its transatlantic form[15] but was not accepted by the majority of the Lords in Sidaway. In essence, the standard depends on disclosure of *material information* and the test is satisfied by asking the question: what information would the reasonably prudent patient consider significant in deciding whether or not to agree to treatment?

Although this standard was rejected in Sidaway there is some evidence that the court will be prepared to disregard professional opinion in recognition of the patient's right to material information.[16] The courts have always maintained that they remain the ultimate arbiter of whether or not a legal duty of care has been satisfied and to this end they are not obligated to follow professional opinion, a view recently reiterated in Bolitho.[17] Divergence from the Bolam principle is allowed where the court is not persuaded that the professional opinion is a reasonably held opinion. In respect of the duty of disclosure the courts have been persuaded that professional opinion supporting non-disclosure of risks was not substantiated by the medical evidence and was consequently out of date.[18] Additionally, those for whom disclosure is normal practice cannot invoke the Bolam principle if on any occasion they should omit to do so. They would not be able to rely on professional opinion that supported non-disclosure, because Bolam is for those who lag behind the times and not for those who know better.[19]

Understanding

If the basis of the duty of disclosure is to give a patient the opportunity to make an 'informed choice', then this can only be achieved if the patient is able to understand the information. There is evidence that patients fail to appreciate the significance of information given to them.[20] This is an important aspect of 'informed consent' that is often overlooked or glossed over and probably concerns itself more with the process of disclosure and communication than with the law. It seems, however, that the law has included this part of the process within the duty.

When recommending a particular type of surgery or treatment, the doctor, when warning of the risks, must take reasonable care to ensure that his explanation of the risks is intelligible to his particular patient. The doctor should use language, simple but not misleading, which the doctor perceives from what knowledge and acquaintanceship that he may have of the patient (which may be slight), will be understood by the patient so that the patient can make an informed decision as to whether or not to consent to the recommended surgery or treatment.[18]

Veracity

There can be no doubt that veracity is fundamental to the patient relationship, which is a relationship founded on trust. Quite clearly in any discussion about treatment and options the patient would expect to be told the truth and any consent based on deceit would not be a true consent.

There is, of course, one recognised exception this rule and that is 'therapeutic privilege' where it is felt that the disclosure of certain information would be detrimental to the patient's well-being. Considerable debate surrounds 'therapeutic privilege' and it is expected to be limited to most exceptional circumstances and it is extremely unlikely to be applicable to the provision of dental treatment.

Veracity is important when 'informed consent' is viewed by the healthcare professional as a ritual to protect against later liability. There are, within dentistry, examples of disclosure of risks on a general probability. Warning of a risk of inferior dental nerve dysaesthesia following removal of lower wisdom teeth to conform with 'accepted practice' is not being truthful if in fact the apices of the tooth are (say) 8 mm from the ID canal.[21] Such information is therefore not helpful to the patient in deciding whether to continue with occasional pericoronitis or have the wisdom tooth removed. Indeed, should a patient decide on the basis of this information not to have the tooth removed, he or she cannot be said to have given an 'informed refusal' and the dentist may liable for the continued suffering for failing to provide adequate advice.

Conclusion

The greater part of this chapter on 'informed consent' has concentrated on the legal aspects of the doctrine, but that does not lessen the importance of the 'doctrine' as a moral concept. It probably reflects the emphasis given to it, and the concerns attached to it, by the profession. Viewed from the legal perspective, it tends to be regarded as an endpoint following the disclosure of information, an agreement by the patient to allow a particular treatment made on the basis of a legal minimum of information. To satisfy this legal duty, 'informed consent' is sometimes no more than, and is often expressed as, giving a warning of inherent risks.

As a moral concept the doctrine is more of a process in which there is a two-way exchange of information in order to help the dentist understand the patient's needs and expectations and to help the patient, by providing him/her with information that he or she requires to make a decision about care: to decide whether to accept the treatment offered, choose an alternative or, when there is no choice, to be aware of potential problems and lastly to decline any treatment offered. Such communication is essential to support the principle of patient autonomy and self-determination.

The relationship between the two perspectives is no better put than by Beauchamp and Childress:

> Legal and professional rules of disclosure should only serve to initiate the communication process, and professionals and their institutions should not be satisfied with a signed consent form unless attention has also been paid to the process that led to it.[22]

References and notes

1 Slater v Baker & Stephenson [1767] *2 Wils KB* 360. The court held that it was reasonable that a patient be told what is about to be done to him so that he may take courage.
2 Harris J (1988) *The Value of Life*. Routledge, London.
3 Which presumably includes no treatment and the consequences of that.
4 Health Service Circular, HSC1999/031. NHS Executive, Leeds.
5 Kennedy I and Grubb A (1994) *Medical Law: text with materials*. Butterworths, London.
6 Cole v Turner [1704] *6 Mod* 149.
7 Wilson v Pringle [1986] *2 All ER* 440. The court attempted to introduce a requirement of hostility into the tort of trespass.
8 Wilding v Lambert Southwark & Lewisham AHA [1982] (unreported).
9 Re T (adult: refusal of medical treatment) [1992] *4 All ER* 649.
10 Chatterton v Gerson [1981] *1 All ER* 257 per Bristow at 265.
11 Sidaway v Board of Governors of the Royal Bethlem Hospital and the Maudsley Hospital [1985] *1 All ER* 643.
12 Maynard v West Midlands RHA [1984] *1 WLR* 634.
13 Whitehouse v Jordan [1981] *1 All ER* 267.
14 Bolam v Friern Hospital Management Committee [1957] *2 All ER* 118 per McNair J at 122.

15 Canterbury v Spence [1972] *464 F.2d 772*. This standard is applied in less than half of the states in America, the majority of states using the 'professional standard'.
16 This view was expressed in Sidaway by Lord Bridge at 505.
17 Bolitho v City and Hackney Health Authority [1997] *4 All ER 771*.
18 Smith v Tunbridge Wells Health Authority [1994] *5 Med LR 334*. Failure to warn of possibility of impotence and bladder dysfunction following surgery for prolapsed rectum. Such a warning would clearly be important to a 28-year-old man.
19 Newell v Goldenberg [1995] *6 Med Lr 371*.
20 Wade TT (1990) Patients may not recall the risk of death: implications for informed consent. *Med Sci Law*. **30**: 259. Only 54% of patients undergoing elective cholecystectomy recalled being told of the risk of death.
21 Any injury resulting would be iatrogenic in origin and not inherent in the procedure.
22 Beauchamp T and Childress J (1994) *Principles of Biomedical Ethics* (4e). Oxford University Press, Oxford.

CHAPTER NINE

Dental care for children

Jenny King

You are the bows from which your children as living arrows are sent forth.
(Kahlil Gibran, *The Prophet*)

This chapter will explore how the ethical and legal considerations that govern dentistry apply in childhood. Most dental care for children is carried out without difficulty and – perhaps contrary to adult expectations – children are very good dental patients. However, moral dilemmas may sometimes arise which may be difficult to resolve. On the one hand there is the need to protect the child's welfare by providing necessary care and on the other hand there is the need to respect another person's right to refuse that care. There is a moral tension between the dangers of either neglect or abuse. It is essential that dentists have the highest standards of professional practice when providing dental care for those who are vulnerable and immature. An understanding of the law and reflection on the ethical consideration of proxy decision making will help to make sure that dental care for children is provided in a mutually acceptable way.

Childhood

Childhood extends from infancy to adolescence. It is a crucial time of growth and development, physically, intellectually and emotionally. Throughout childhood a person is to a greater or lesser extent dependent on others for basic support, most often from their parents. As childhood progresses a child becomes increasingly independent until adult maturity is reached.

Dental problems are common and the two major plaque-related diseases, dental decay and gum disease, can both start in childhood. There may also be accidents to teeth and orthodontic treatment for malocclusions is itself a specialty within dentistry. Children are encouraged to attend the dentist regularly from the age of three onwards or even earlier. Over a quarter of the patients registered with General Dental Services in England are children.[1]

Childhood is a time of vulnerability since children do not have the full capacity to make choices for themselves. Children may have little say in life events, even though they directly concern them, leaving them feeling that they lack any control over what happens to them. But growing up is a process of learning to be a self-determining person and an essential part of parenting is to nurture a child's evolving autonomy. Those adults providing professional care have similar responsibilities to respect and promote children's autonomy. This means that children's capacity to make their own decisions should be encouraged whilst at the same time receiving needful adult support.

A child's maturity will depend on many factors and no two children will be the same, but all children, of whatever age, deserve such consideration whether it is in the home, in the school or in the clinic. In the provision of healthcare doctors and dentists have an important moral as well as legal responsibility towards child patients to acknowledge their vulnerability and to respect them as developing persons.[2]

Ethical and legal considerations

Although the age of majority in the United Kingdom is 18, the legal age at which a person can consent to medical treatment was set at 16 in 1969 in the Family Law Reform Act.[3] For a child below the age of 16 the law requires the consent of a parent or person with parental responsibility before any treatment is carried out although there may be some circumstances where children under 16 can consent without parental involvement. This is accepted in England and Wales and in many other countries. Even the natural father who is not married to the child's mother cannot take parental responsibility unless he has been made a legal guardian or there is parental agreement.

However, the Children Act 1989 section 3(5) states that any person who has charge of a child may do 'what is reasonable in all the circumstances of the case for the purpose of safeguarding or promoting the child's welfare'. This could include dental treatment. However, although emergency or routine treatment might be included irreversible procedures would require the consent of a person with parental responsibility.[4] In emergency situations, therefore, a child can at times be treated without a parent's knowledge or consent. A dental example might be replacing a front tooth which has been knocked out in an accident at school, where delay would reduce the likelihood of successful reimplantation. In this situation the dentist acts in the child's best interest and indeed it might be considered negligent not to do so.[3]

In recent years there has been an increasing emphasis on the rights that children themselves have. This has been outlined in the United Nations Convention on the Rights of the Child which states in relation to health that children have a right to 'the enjoyment of the highest attainable standard of health and facilities for the treatment of illness'.[5] In England and Wales the Children Act recognises that a child has the right to be consulted about his or her healthcare.[6] Children should have their dental care explained to them as well as their parents and their views taken into account. In this way a child is able to be involved in decisions about their dental treatment whilst at the same time parents and other adults continue to give them the support that they still require.

The accepted ethical principles to protect life and health, respect autonomy and to do so justly and fairly[7] apply to parents and children as well as to adults. Consent should be based on information, comprehension and be freely given and information should be given about the child's dental condition, treatment options, including no treatment, and any risks and benefits.[8] The rules of privacy in receiving dental treatment also extend to parents and children. Confidentiality should be maintained and no information should be given to a third party unless consent has first been obtained. This means, for example, that a schoolteacher does not have any right to information about a child's dental treatment or dental attendance. It also means that parents should not be given information about dental care which a competent young person asks to remain private.

Children of different ages

The level at which any child has the capacity to be involved in decisions about their dental care will depend to some extent on how old they are, although chronological age is by no means the only factor and culture and education also play an important part. For instance, a three year old who requires a general anaesthetic for the extraction of a painful molar is less likely to take part in the decisions than a teenager receiving orthodontic treatment who is likely to be very involved in treatment decisions.

Although 16 is set as the age at which a person can consent for themselves, the law does make provision for younger children of sufficient maturity who expressly do not wish to involve their parents. This follows the landmark case in 1985 of Gillick v West Norfolk and Wisbech AHA where an underage teenager requested contraceptive advice.[3] The judgement was eventually made that children under 16 could receive medical care without their parent's consent if the doctor judged them to be mature enough to reason about and comprehend their care. This ruling has general application, including to dental treatment, and has led to the concept known as 'Gillick competence'.

This is an important recognition that 16 is an arbitrary age and that there is a need for some flexibility. Again, however, parental consent will normally be sought for adolescents. It is only in exceptional circumstances when a child is unable to or refuses to involve their parents and necessary treatment cannot otherwise go ahead that the law allows the child themselves to give consent for the dentist to proceed if they are judged to be mature enough to do so.

Some writers have argued that children can consent for themselves at a much earlier age, whilst acknowledging that parents should continue to give them support. Alderson,[9] for example, in her study of children undergoing surgery, suggests that experience of receiving healthcare is something that helps children to develop their own decision-making capabilities long before they reach the age of 16. This reinforces the principle that children are persons in their own right. As one eight year old reported in a recent study of consent in dental care: 'I'd rather be involved because it's me they're doing it to'.[10]

Although a parent must sign any consent form some practitioners have introduced the idea of child assent as a way of involving the child as well. In this case the form is signed jointly, the parent consents and the child assents to be treated.[11]

The management of child patients

Proper explanation plays an important part in patient management. For instance, in the study of consent in dental care children who had previously been uncooperative for dental treatment explained how being more involved helped them to be able to cope better. One father explained how his son had been so upset at the dentist that he had resorted to violence and given his mother a black eye. However, when he had things explained to him this enabled him to receive the dental treatment that he needed.[10] This illustrates how knowing about treatment can help children to co-operate.

The fact that dentists now often examine and treat children, especially younger children, with parents present in the surgery is an advantage in that explanations are given to everyone and it is not necessary to repeat information to parents later. This allows parents and children together to consider the options and be involved in choices about the way in which treatment might be managed. Involvement creates a greater trust and confidence for children, parents and dentists.

Most children are able to accept dental treatment which may at times be quite complex and uncomfortable. Proper attention to explanations and pain control can make difficult situations manageable for all concerned. However, there are occasions when children do refuse to co-operate with dental treatment. In the past children have been forced to have treatment that dentists and parents considered was in their best interests. However, guidelines from the General Dental Council are quite clear that treatment should not be forced on unwilling children. They suggest that it is better to wait and arrange a further appointment.

> There can be no justification for intimidation or, other than in the most exceptional circumstance, for the use of physical restraint in dealing with a difficult patient. When faced with a child who is uncontrollable for whatever reason the dentist should consider ceasing treatment, making an appropriate explanation to the parent ... and arranging necessary future treatment for the child rather than continuing in these circumstances.[12]

Although a dentist may obtain legal consent from parents to treat a child and may thereby proceed even against the child's will, there remains a moral responsibility towards the child patient. This is an illustration of how legal and ethical standards may not always agree. In the long term there is little to be gained by forcing treatment on an unwilling child. Respect for children will ultimately depend not on the law but on the willingness of dentists to involve child patients in decisions about their care.

As Montgomery suggests: 'The extent to which young people will actually be denied the chance to decide what health care they receive is in the hands of the health care professionals who care for them'.[13]

Children can consent to medical treatment when they are 16 but at present the law in England does not allow them to refuse treatment until they are 18. Many of the recent cases that have come to court have concerned anorexic teenagers and decisions about forced feeding, as in re W, a minor, 1992.[6] However, there could be occasions when a 17 year old refuses dental treatment against the wishes of his/her parents. Since dental problems are rarely life threatening and most dental treatment is elective there is the possibility of leaving any treatment until children are old enough to decide for themselves. Although a person may not wish to co-operate at the time he or she may well be more likely to accept treatment later in life in the knowledge that the right to accept or to refuse treatment was respected.

If children are in voluntary care then their parents' consent for dental treatment should be sought. For children who are subject to a care order social services may have parental responsibility for consent to dental care. However, it is always good practice to involve parents as well if possible, particularly if dental treatment is serious, such as for extractions or general anaesthesia.

There may be occasions when parents speak little English and have only limited understanding of dentistry. Sometimes the child him or herself or an older sibling may act as an informal interpreter. But where the dental situation is complex, for example the long-term management of treatment for a child with a cleft palate or a serious complicating medical condition, a bilingual health advocate is essential before embarking on treatment.

There may sometimes be disagreements between the parents about a child's dental care; for instance, a mother and father may disagree about the advisability of fissure sealants. Although the law requires the consent of only one parent[13] in this instance, since treatment is elective, it is possible to defer any decision until parents can come to their own agreement. Sometimes a dentist may suggest a treatment with which parents disagree, for example extracting other carious teeth if a general anaesthetic is required, whilst a parent may want only the one tooth causing pain to be extracted. Although efforts should always be made to take time to explain and negotiate it is only legally acceptable to do the treatment to which parents have consented, even if the dentist believes that an alternative treatment would be better for the child. However, dentists have no legal obligation to carry out treatment which they believe would not be in the child's best interests.

In the past dental treatment for young children has often been the extraction of decayed primary teeth under general anaesthesia in dental practice. But improving dental health and the risk of morbidity or even mortality have resulted in far fewer dental anaesthetics for children. The latest guidelines from the General Dental Council[12] require that general anaesthetics are only given under specialist care and with access to hospital resuscitation and emergency care. It is the responsibility of the referring practitioner to justify to parents the necessity for a general anaesthetic. General anaesthesia for dental treatment for children should only be used when other possibilities have been thoroughly explored and it should not be used as a substitute for good communication and patient management skills.

Patience, discussion and negotiation with parents and children as well as consultation with dental colleagues should be able to resolve the problems which arise when treating children. In persistently difficult situations children may be referred to a specialist hospital department. National dental bodies such as the British Dental Association and the defence organisations will also give advice. Only in very rare circumstances in dentistry should there be any necessity to refer a case to the family court but this remains a possibility.

Child abuse

Occasionally a dentist may notice evidence of trauma to a child which raises a suspicion of physical abuse. Broken or lost teeth or facial bruising may suggest that the child has been hit. In infancy there may be trauma where a dummy has been forcibly pushed into a baby's mouth. These situations are not easy to deal with but health authorities have local policies for reporting suspicious injuries. The dentist would not normally deal directly with such a situation but should first contact the child's general medical practitioner or seek advice from the local health authority. A dentist may be seen as a trusted adult and a child may confide in them about sexual abuse. Reporting should be the same as for physical abuse but it is important to negotiate very sensitively with the child about the need to report it. [3,14]

Aggressive medical treatment may itself become abusive. [15] Physical punishment such as smacking is never appropriate in the provision of healthcare. Many adults can trace dental phobias to unpleasant experiences in childhood. Poor management can leave a legacy of fear which may be very difficult to overcome in later years. Restraining techniques have been used to carry out treatment on the ground that it is for a child's own good. Techniques such as the hand over mouth exercise (HOME) are still being described in dental textbooks, especially in North America. [16] Such restraint is in danger of being both abusive and counterproductive.

Relationships between dentists, parents and children

Good management techniques which take time to familiarise the child and their parents with the dental environment and involve them by explaining rather than forcing treatment are more likely to be successful in achieving children's co-operation and in establishing long-term acceptance of dental treatment. The increasing emphasis on the prevention of disease and the reduction in levels of dental decay in western societies have made dental care for children much more manageable in recent years.

Consider the case of eight-year-old Becky who comes into the surgery with her mother and father. This is her first dental visit. She has been kept awake with a painful tooth. Examination shows that she has several decayed teeth and that a lower right primary molar is causing the present pain. Her first permanent molars are present but as yet do not have any decay. Becky is crying and climbing out of the dental chair. The dentist's immediate thought is to write a brief referral letter to the local hospital for this tooth to be extracted with a general anaesthetic. On the other hand it would almost certainly be possible to restore the tooth. The dentist decides to tell the family about the options and explains how the toothache can be controlled with analgesics and a simple dressing. She explains about introducing Becky slowly to dental care so that she becomes familiar with the dental environment before starting treatment. She also mentions about prevention in the future. In this situation explaining the options and offering choices helps people to understand and own the decisions that are made, increasing the likelihood of co-operation whichever option is finally decided upon.

Unlike the one-to-one relationships that dentists have with adult patients, in children's dentistry at least three people are involved. It can be seen from the discussion so far that good professional practice in treating children depends on the establishment of good relationships between dentists and children and their parents. This requires dentists to have an understanding of moral and legal principles and to have developed the necessary professional skills to apply them in practice. This might be summed up in the principle of 'tell, show and do'.

The latest educational guidance from the GDC lays new emphasis on the importance of including ethics and law and communication skills in the dental curriculum. Knowledge attitudes and skills in relation to these aspects of dentistry are as important in dental education as learning the necessary technical clinical skills.[17,18] Making decisions on behalf of another person, particularly when that person is young and vulnerable, is not easy for adult dentists and parents.[19] But it can be made easier by being honest and open with children and their parents, taking time to provide information and explanations in a child-friendly way. People are less likely to feel anxious when they feel in control of their situation. This will help to establish confidence in the dental profession from an early age. Furthermore, good care in childhood will help people to accept treatment more easily in adult life and reduce some of the anxiety and stress which has been associated with dentistry.

Conclusion

The ethical and legal responsibility to respect children as well as those who support them is essential in establishing good professional relationships. Understanding of the moral significance of childhood and the responsibility of adults to protect and nurture children without compulsion is not an optional extra but an integral part of good dentistry. Good communication will be rewarded with healthier smiles from children and their parents.

References and notes

1   *Health and Personal Social Services Statistics for England 1997*. HMSO, London.
2   Ozar D and Sokol D (1994) *Dental Ethics at Chairside*. Mosby, St Louis.
3   Brazier M (1993) *Medicine, Patients and the Law*. Penguin, Harmondsworth.
4   Bainham A (1998) *Children: the modern law*. Family Law, Bristol.
5   United Nations Convention on the Rights of the Child 1989 Article 24.
6   McHale J and Fox M (1997) *Health Care Law*. Sweet and Maxwell, London.
7   Beauchamp T and Childress J (1994) *Principles of Biomedical Ethics*. Oxford University Press, New York.
8   Faden R and Beauchamp T (1986) *A History and Theory of Informed Consent*. Oxford University Press, New York.
9   Alderson P (1993) *Childrens' Consent to Surgery*. Open University Press, Buckingham.
10 King J, Hillier S and Doyal L (2000) *Consent in Dental Care*. King's Fund, London.
11 Mouradian W (1999) Making decisions for children. *Angle Orthod.* **69**(4): 300–5.
12 General Dental Council (1997) *Maintaining Standards*. GDC, London.
13 Montgomery J (1997) *Health Care Law*. Oxford University Press, Oxford.
14 Welbury R and Murphy J (1998) The dental practitioner's role in protecting children from abuse. *Br Dental J.* **184**(3): 115–19.
15 Doyal L (1998) Can medicine be torture? In: G Van Bueren (ed) *Childhood Abused*. Ashgate, Aldershot.
16 McDonald R and Avery D (2000) *Dentistry for the Child and Adolescent*. Mosby, St Louis.
17 General Dental Council (1997) *The First Five Years*. GDC, London.
18 Bridgman A, Collier A, Cunningham J *et al.* (1999) Teaching and assessing ethics and law in the dental curriculum. *Br Dental J.* **187**(4): 217–19.
19 Buchanan A and Brock D (1989) *Deciding for Others*. Cambridge University Press, Cambridge.

CHAPTER TEN

Mentally disabled adults: a vulnerable group

Andrew Bridgman

Introduction

The treatment of adult patients with a mental disability can often present the dentist with a variety of complex and perplexing problems. Perhaps the most difficult question arising from the disability will be the patient's capability to participate in treatment decisions. The effect of the disability on mental capacity is not necessarily an 'all-or-nothing' phenomenon and the patient may or may not be capable of making decisions about treatment.

The matter may be further complicated by the patient's behaviour. The patient may be non-communicative. Is such behaviour an outward manifestation of their illness or arrested development or do they simply not understand? The patient may be compliant and co-operative. Should this co-operation be interpreted as agreement with the treatment? Has such a patient consented or made no decision at all? What about the patient who actively resists attempts at treatment, perhaps even when it is clear that they are suffering with toothache? Is such behaviour indicative that the patient does not want treatment? Is it a decision that ought to be respected or is it no decision at all? The potential exists, particularly in the last example, for conflict between the ethical principles of helping those who are in need of help and recognising their right to make their own decisions.

Mental disability

The World Health Organization has described disability as a functional limitation arising from physical, intellectual or sensory impairment, medical conditions or mental illness. The Mental Health Act 1983 does not define mental disability but a recent policy statement, *Making Decisions*, outlining the government's proposal for reform in this area of law, gives a clear definition. It defines mental disability as 'any disability or disorder of the mind or brain, whether permanent or temporary, which results in an impairment or disturbance of mental functioning'.[1] The term 'mental disability' can therefore be used to describe all groups of patients so affected, but there are important differences that depend on the cause of the disability. Those groups of patients often referred to as having 'learning difficulties' have a disability that is congenital in origin or caused by disease or trauma as a child. They have an incomplete or arrested development, they may have never reached full capacity and because of this they may be limited in their decision-making ability. This can make assessment difficult because of their lack of previously held values or views.

Patients who acquire their disability in adult life cannot be described as having a learning difficulty. It may be presumed that at one time they were of full capacity which has now been diminished because of pathological processes or physical injury. Making an assessment for this group of patients is sometimes easier because they will have previously held values.

The combination of an ageing population, increasing prevalence of dementia, people with 'learning difficulties' living longer and a philosophy of care within the community will result in many more patients with some degree of mental disability requesting treatment from the general dental services or the community dental services.

Assessment of competence

Competence is defined as the ability to perform a task, in this instance to make a decision. In this sense competence is recognised as a specific rather than global concept, even though there is a presumption that all adult patients are competent to make decisions for themselves. However, where there is evidence of mental disability this is a presumption that can be rebutted but it is important to remember that mental disability does not equate with incompetence. The attending dentist must therefore make a thorough assessment of the patient's decisional capacity. A thorough and documented assessment is essential, primarily to protect the rights of a vulnerable member of society, rights which are supported in law and of particular importance when the patient appears to be refusing treatment. It would be a trespass to treat such a patient if the refusal is valid. It would be negligent to deny care if the refusal was not valid because the law has established a common law duty to provide care for those patients disabled from giving consent.[2]

The assessment of competence should follow a 'functional approach' which would depend on whether the patient is able at the time to understand the nature and effect of their decision.[1] Clearly such a test focuses on *ability* to understand[3] but other criteria are important adjuncts to this assessment. In what is regarded as a seminal paper Roth *et al.*[4] identified and described five tests for the assessment of competence:

- evidencing a choice
- reasonable outcome of choice
- choice based on rational reasons
- ability to understand information
- actual understanding of information.

These tests cannot, however, stand in isolation from each other and consideration of their interdependence has provided the essence of much discussion.[5]

Based on the presumption that all adult patients have the capacity to make decisions for themselves, expression of their choice will satisfy the test of competence. It is the lowest level test for competence and the test that is most respectful of patient autonomy. It would not matter that the outcome of their choice is not reasonable in the opinion of others or that the reasons for their decision are irrational.

After all:

> [t]housands of patients whose competence is never questioned stay away from dentists out of 'irrational fear' to the detriment of their dental, and sometimes their general, health.[6]

It is only when there is doubt about the patient's ability to understand that questions of competency arise. Such doubts may emerge where the patient has a mental disability and the choice that is being made does not have a reasonable outcome and/or it appears not to be based on rational reasons. An example might be a 72-year-old man with moderate dementia who is thought to be suffering toothache yet actively, and perhaps fiercely, resists attempts at examination. In this situation the dentist will be alerted to the possibility of incompetence and will need to determine whether or not the patient is capable of understanding the nature and effect of his decision. It is an important assessment to make, the measure of which cannot be overestimated. Without assessing the validity of the 'refusal' the dentist will be in danger of either over-riding the patient's rights of self-determination, if he continues with treatment despite the objections, or failing to help the patient, if he accepts the 'refusal' at face value.

The functional approach to an assessment based on ability to understand will probably involve others in the process, although responsibility lies with the attending dentist. The views of family and carers are important to the assessment process but a recent study showed a range of attitudes to the decision-making capacity of patients with mental disability, falling into four broad categories.

1   Recognising that the patient had the right to make choices and support- ing him/her to do so.
2   Assuming the person had no preference and would simply acquiesce with whatever was decided on his/her behalf.
3   Accepting that the person was expressing a preference but deeming that preference to be 'wrong' or 'misguided'.
4   Thinking the person was unable to make any choice.[7]

A dentist needs to take into account the views of others but should do so with caution.

A test that bases itself on ability to understand has the advantage that it allows the dentist to broaden the process, away from dental treatment, to include discussions of more general matters and other aspects of the patient's everyday living. Such an approach must also endorse the belief that com- petency or the ability to understand is dependent on the ability to process information rationally, that the choice is based on a set of enduring values[8] or that it reflects the value the patient would have previously given to the benefit (or detriment) of treatment.[9] The law appears to support this belief.[10]

It might be the case that a patient, now with senile dementia, had only sought dental treatment when absolutely necessary. If that is so, then the behaviour described in the above example might be indicative of a valid refusal. On the other hand, if the patient had previously been a regular attender for whom dental health was important, then resistance would seem inconsistent with those values. In this situation resistance is more likely to be indicative of a lack of understanding.

Treatment without consent

Treatment without consent is a battery (commonly called assault) in the tort of trespass of the person and in the criminal law (Chapter 7). For patients below the age of 18 who lack the capacity to give consent to treatment, it is possible to obtain proxy consent. However, in the case of adult patients, despite misconceptions to the contrary, no such proxy consent is available either at common law or under the Mental Health Act 1983.[11] The govern- ment's proposals for statutory reform of the law include the introduction of proxy consent either from a wider Continuing Power of Attorney[1] or from a court-appointed manager.[1] However, legislative change is probably 3–4 years away.

Therefore an assessment that a patient lacks the necessary capacity to consent to or refuse treatment creates the problem that any treatment provided will be *prima facie* unlawful.

Lawful treatment

In 1989, the House of Lords addressed the untenable position of healthcare professionals being liable for battery if they treated a patient incapable of giving consent.[2] The House, itself unable to give lawful consent,[12] determined that it had the power to make a declaration that the operation would be lawful. However, it concluded that such a declaration would not be necessary, for any proposed operation or treatment would be lawful provided that it could be considered, in the circumstances, to be in the best interests of the patient.

> In common law a doctor can lawfully operate on or give other treatment to adult patients who are incapable of consenting to his doing so, provided that the operation or treatment is in the best interests of such patients. The operation will be in their best interests only if it is carried out in order either to save their lives or to ensure improvement or prevent deterioration in their physical or mental health.[2]

The second part of the 'best interests' test clearly gives scope for a broad range of interventions and authority to all responsible for the care of such patients.

Best interests test

Providing treatment that is considered to be in the best interests of the patient, in situations where they are unable to consent, is justified by the doctrine of necessity which in essence arises from the inability to communicate with the 'assisted person'. That inability may arise because there is insufficient time if any action to be taken is going to prevent injury or possible death or because the 'assisted person' is unable to communicate, either because he or she is unconscious or because of a mental disability.

It is important to distinguish between application of the doctrine and 'best interests' where the ability to communicate is temporarily absent, such as the emergency situation of unconsciousness or general anaesthesia, and where it is lost permanently.[2] In the former the actions taken should be no more than is reasonably required to return the patient to a state of well-being, to a state of consciousness that will allow him or her to make decisions about further treatment. Where the patient is never going to be in a position to make such decisions or be involved in the process, then the doctrine extends to embrace that need for care which is obvious, including: 'such humdrum matters as routine medical or dental treatment, even simple care such as dressing and undressing, and putting to bed'.[2] 'Simple care' is an important addendum to the test because battery is not limited to medical and dental care but applies to any non-consensual touching.

The doctrine of necessity has its origins in mercantile law and is conditional upon the satisfaction of two conditions. The treatment of those incapable of providing consent requires the same conditions to be fulfilled. First, there must be a necessity to act in circumstances when it is not possible to obtain the patient's agreement. Second, the action taken must be one which a reasonable person would have taken, in the circumstances, in the best interests of the assisted person.[2]

In relation to healthcare the actions of a reasonable person would usually be interpreted as the actions of a reasonable doctor or dentist and that also applies to the best interests test. Regard would be paid to that treatment which a reasonable body of medical/dental opinion would consider appropriate. Whether or not the treatment provided was in the best interests of the patient is a professionally determined test, imported from the tort of negligence, as laid out in Bolam[2] (see Chapter 12).

The use of restraint

Sometimes patients who lack the capacity to make valid decisions put up fierce resistance against attempts at treatment or even an examination. For care to be provided safely, for both the patient and the dental team, the patient's behaviour will need to be controlled using some means of restraint: physical force, sedation or general anaesthesia.

The lawfulness of the use of restraint was not considered in F v West Berkshire, although some legal commentators believe that it was implicit in the judgement.[13] It was some years before a court of authority explored the lawful use of restraint. In a case involving a Caesarean section, the Court of Appeal affirmed the opinion that it formed part of the best interests test and was therefore a clinical judgement.[14] As such, the lawfulness of the use of restraint will, in all likelihood, be judged according to the professional standard as laid down in Bolam. It is important to remember, however, that the judiciary retains the privilege of being the ultimate arbiter of whether or not that professional opinion is responsible or reasonably held.[15]

Research

Although the ethical and legal aspects of research in general are covered in Chapter 14 there are important considerations specific to this vulnerable group of society.

In essence, the lawfulness of research on the human subject is governed by the common law requirements of consent. It might seem, therefore, that the principles applicable to treatment would also apply to research. That is not so.

The introduction to this chapter talked about the non-communicative but compliant and co-operative patient. Is this patient consenting to treatment or making no decision? In so far as treatment is concerned, it does not matter. The dentist is able to proceed lawfully either on the basis of the patient's consent or in accordance with the best interests test. The dentist is able to proceed in the apparent absence of the patient's consent. This approach might be available to the researcher for therapeutic research, provided that there is absolutely true equipoise in the trial. The researcher must remember that he/she has a duty to act in the *best interests* of the patient. Thus much will depend on the nature of the research and the amount of information that the patient will have to understand. If there are concerns there must be a clear consent from the patient; mere absence of dissent will not suffice.

The legal position where the research is non-therapeutic is more uncertain. Non-therapeutic research by its definition will not directly benefit the research subject but because it is carried out to advance understanding of the illness or disability, the patient may ultimately benefit.

Obtaining consent for research may be more complex than obtaining consent for treatment and the ethical outlook may be ahead of the law in this respect. All ethical guidelines suggest that subjects must be fully informed before agreeing to participate in research. This requires that they are aware of the nature and purpose of the research, the benefits to be gained either for them or advancement of knowledge, the risks and possible side effects and discomfort. The duty to give such advice (informed consent) is seemingly determined by a 'reasonable patient (person) standard' rather than the 'professional standard' in relation to treatment. This will require that research subjects demonstrate a greater level of understanding if their agreement to participate is accepted than if they are patients consenting to treatment. In research involving human subjects the patients' interests are secondary to the quest for knowledge; they are a means to an end and it is right that the requirements for consent are more rigorous, even if this means that many adults lacking capacity will be barred from participating in research trials.

The Declaration of Helsinki[16] states: 'In case of legal incompetence, informed consent should be obtained from the legal guardian in accordance with national legislation'. UK law does not, however, allow proxy consent for adults. Ethical guidance,[17] on the other hand, suggests that research involving such subjects would be ethical following discussion with relatives and scrutiny of the project by an independent body.[18] The law supports discussion with family when deciding to provide treatment as 'it may reveal information as to the personal circumstances of the patient and as to the choice the patient might have made, if he or she had been in a position to make it'.[19] Such discussion would be equally helpful in deciding whether a person would have agreed to being involved in research, either therapeutic or non-therapeutic. However, as with treatment, it is only a helpful adjunct if that person has at one time been in a position to make such a decision. It would not apply to a person with severe learning difficulties. Whether or not the law at present would accept ethical guidelines as the basis for lawful research on adults lacking the capacity to decide for themselves is uncertain.

Ethical guidelines also suggest that the use of vulnerable groups as research subjects, for example children and adults without capacity, should be avoided if the same results can be acquired using 'normal adults'. In so far as research in dentistry is concerned it would seem unlikely that adults lacking capacity could provide any different results and their use as research subjects would be exceptional.

Conclusion

Adults with a mental disability are vulnerable members of society. There is the danger that because of their disability they will be labelled as incompetent and deemed unable to participate in any decision-making process. They will be denied their right of self-determination. On the other hand, however, too much emphasis on their 'right to choose' may deny them the help that they require, if they lack the capacity to exercise that right.

The provision of healthcare for this group of patients illustrates the fragility of the relationship between concern for the patient as a person (and respect for their autonomy) and concern for their welfare. Great care must be exercised when attending such patients.

References and notes

1   Department of Health (1999) *Making Decisions*. HMSO, London.
2   F v West Berkshire HA [1989] *2 All ER* 545.
3   Re MB [1997] *8 Med LR* 217; Health Service Circular, HSC 1999/031.
4   Roth L, Meisel A and Lidz C (1977) Tests of competency to consent to treatment. *Am J Psychiatry*. **134**: 279–84.
5   Beauchamp T and Childress J (1994) *Principles of Biomedical Ethics*. Oxford University Press, New York; Appelbaum P and Grisso T (1998) Assessing patient's capacities to consent to treatment. *New Engl J Med*. **319**: 1635–8; Buchanan A and Brock D (1989) *Deciding for Others*. Cambridge University Press, Cambridge; Gunn M (1994) The meaning of capacity. *Med Law Rev*. **2**: 8–29; Wicclair M (1991) Patient decision making capacity and risk. *Bioethics*. **5**: 118–22.
6   Brazier M (1991) Competence, consent and proxy consents. In: M Brazier and M Lobjoit (eds) *Protecting the Vulnerable*. Routledge, London.
7   Stalker K, Duckett P and Downs M (1991) *Going with the Flow: choice, dementia and people with learning difficulties*. Joseph Rowntree Foundation, Pavilion Publishing, London.
8   Buchanan A and Brock D (1989) *Deciding for Others*. Cambridge University Press, Cambridge.
9   Appelbaum P and Grisso T (1988) Assessing patients' capabilities to consent to treatment. *New Engl J Med*. **319**: 1635–8.
10   R v Blaue [1975] *3 All ER* 446; Re T (adult: refusal of medical treatment) [1992] *4 All ER* 649.
11   T v T and another [1988] *1 All ER* 613; F v West Berkshire HA [1989] *2 All ER* 545.
12   The courts' jurisdiction over adults of unsound mind was lost with revocation of the Warrant assigned to the Lord Chancellor and the judges of the High Court and the enactment of the Mental Health Act 1959, both events taking place on 1 November 1960.
13   Grubb A (1994) Treatment without consent (anorexia nervosa) adult. *Med Law Rev*. **2**: 95–9.
14   Re MB [1997] *8 Med LR* 217. For further discussion see Bridgman AM and Wilson MA (2000) The treatment of adult patients with mental disability. Part 3: The use of restraint. *Br Dental J*. **189**: 195–8.
15   Bolitho v City and Hackney HA [1997] 4 *All ER* 771.
16   *Recommendation Guiding Medical Doctors in Biomedical Research Involving Human Subjects* (revised 1975). Paragraph 10.
17   Royal College of Physicians (1990) *Guidelines on the Practice of Ethics Committees in Research Involving Human Subjects*. RCP, London; Royal College of Physicians (1990) *Research Involving Patients*. RCP, London; Royal College of Psychiatrists (1990) Guidelines for the research ethics committees on psychiatric research involving human subjects. *Psych Bull*. **14**: 48–61.
18   As that provided by local research ethics committees.
19   Re T (adult: refusal of medical treatment) [1992] 4 *All ER* 649 per Lord Donaldson at 653.

CHAPTER ELEVEN

Practising in the NHS

Graham Walsh

Establishment of the NHS: moral foundations

> No society can legitimately call itself civilised if a sick person is denied medical aid because of lack of means ...
>
> (Aneurin Bevan, 1941)

The Hippocratic Oath and its modern equivalent is but one of many responses regarding the relationship between doctor and patient. The biblical acclamation, 'I did not know I was my brother's keeper' and the Hindu Carka Samhita of the Hindu Code imply that both eastern and western moral philosophies play a part in the role of the doctor–patient relationship. It relates to a continuum between government and the population and, perhaps contemporaneously, between global organisations and human kind.

The UK is in many ways unique. The origins of its social welfare provisions can be traced to the philosophy of utilitarianism as espoused by Jeremy Bentham (1748–1831) and John Stuart Mill (1836–1873). It was Mill who said: 'Poverty is the parent of a thousand mental and moral ills ... medical care is a basic human need, a healthful community is a basic social need'.

Social deprivation probably reached its apogee at the time of the 1930s depression, the consequence of which was to exclude a large number of the population from social welfare provision. Medical and surgical treatment was provided by a fragmented medical service (panel doctors). Hospitals were either voluntary, supported by charitable funds, or public hospitals, many of which had an air of decrepitude, the result of their conversion from a non-medical function in the Victorian era. Local authorities did provide community care but much depended on the dynamic of the particular local authority.

The genesis of the National Health Service can be located in the deliberations of the Royal Commission on the Poor Law (1905), specifically the

Webbs Minority Report which was, in effect, the basis for state-provided healthcare. It was this burden of despair together with the increasing development of medical and social science that provided the impetus for the formation of an interdepartmental inquiry set up specifically 'on the co-ordination of social insurance'. William Beveridge was to be its chairman.

The Committee on Social Insurance and Allied Services was established in June 1941. This alone was a remarkable exhibition of faith in the future. The Beveridge Report was completed by 1942 but its publication was postponed because some Cabinet members of the wartime coalition government thought it too radical. The Beveridge Report was based on three principles: full employment, family allowances and a universal national health service. Beveridge considered that spending on welfare should be regarded as a social investment and that a universal health service, apart from the moral basis of giving treatment and care to those who needed it, would, by its very nature, produce an increasingly healthy population. It should increase the work output of the population that was much needed for post-war reconstruction.

Ultimately, all resources came from central taxation through the National Insurance stamp, a symbol of the underestimation of demand, but the unique message from the Beveridge Report was that health services should be provided free at the point of delivery. No one should be prevented from receiving treatment that was considered necessary to maintain health and, where dentistry was concerned, to maintain oral health.

Within two years of the start of the National Health Service on 1 July 1948, prescription charges were introduced. Today, as far as dentistry is concerned, some 33% of the gross fees are represented by patient charges.

The changes evoked built on the development of local health authorities, regional hospital boards and executive councils. Doctors and Dentists would be independent contractors to the executive councils. There have been many changes to these arrangements since 1948, principally in 1974, 1988 and 1990 (with the introduction of the purchaser/provider model). The 1990 changes were based on the government White Papers *Working for Patients* and *Promoting Better Health*. Nevertheless, in spite of all the changes that have occurred, the idea of a health service free at the point of delivery survives in part.

The architects of the National Health Service assumed that free health services for all would lead to a drop in demand as treatment needs declined due to a predicted reduction in disease levels. The paradigm for this theory was the drop in the incidence of infectious diseases in the late 1940s and 1950s. This, of course, has not occurred. Instead we have experienced burgeoning demand for the alleviation of chronic illness. This gap between supply and demand has been addressed by an enlarging independent private sector and increasing waiting lists in the public sector. Nevertheless, the ultimate moral basis is the interaction between patient and practitioner and this ethic is embraced by the concept of 'informed consent' and equity of access to care.

The inclusion of evidence-based medicine as a natural philosophy of medicine and the creation of the National Institute for Clinical Excellence are no doubt outcomes of the escalating costs of the health service, but they also embrace the values of healthcare. There is a convergence of both the moral and the scientific basis underpinning the concept of a universal health service.

However, future predictions suggest that within the next 50 years most chronic disease will be preventable and populations will live longer and have an improved quality of life. The elderly will retain their independence for much longer than hitherto, but their ultimate demise will be preceded by a much more rapid deterioration.

Indeed, if these predictions do come true, then Bentham's philosophy of the greatest good for the greatest number of people will have been achieved.

Contractual arrangements

A dentist wishing to provide general dental services in the NHS applies to the health authority in whose area he/she wishes to practise, to be included in the dental list. The health authority checks the applicant's credentials and then submits a form (DTR4) to the Dental Practice Board (DPB) asking for a contract to be opened. This is not a legal contract. The important thing to note is that the 'contract' is the key to obtaining payment for NHS claims; without a valid 'open contract' no payment will be made by the DPB.

Once this form (DTR4) is received by the Dental Contracts section at the DPB, it is recorded and subjected to further detailed checks. The information is then recorded on the DPB mainframe computer which produces a verification print-out which the DPB uses to check and confirm that the appropriate sort of 'contract' has been opened.

The different sorts of 'contract' are as follows.

Single-handed contract

Involves a single dentist as a principal. As such the dentist may have associate dentists working for him/her. However, this type does not involve partners.

Partnership contract

Involves two or more dentists in a percentage-sharing partnership for the provision of general dental services (GDS) or personal dental services (PDS) within a single health authority/pilot PDS area. Each GDS partnership is allocated a unique three-digit number which relates to one address only. If a partnership with two members loses a member it will be dissolved and the DPB should be informed. Partnership contracts may involve the employment of assistants or vocational trainees and may involve associates.

Assistants

An assistant is a qualified dentist employed by another qualified dentist to provide services under the contract number of the employing dentist. The contract number includes the personal number of the principal but uniquely identifies the assistant by means of a suffix. The employing dentist must have at least one single-handed contract at the same address open for the whole time that the contract for the assistant is in force. A dentist may not have more than two assistants or deputies without the consent of the health authority.

If a dentist has a work permit he or she can only work as an employed person, i.e. an assistant to the principal named on the permit. Any amendments to the permit need to be authorised by the Overseas Labour Service. All dentists from abroad who are not from a European Union country or do not have permission from the Home Office require a work permit. The Home Office can give dentists from abroad permission to work in a self-employed status as long as they satisfy certain criteria and have £250 000 to invest in the business. A dentist who has worked for a period of four years with a work permit is able to apply to the Home Office for self-employed status.

Vocational dental practitioner

A vocational trainee/dental practitioner is a newly qualified dentist employed as an assistant by another qualified dentist for a period of training, usually one year. Services are provided by the trainee under the contract number of the employing dentist. Normally, only one trainee may be accommodated for any given contract number. The contract number includes the personal number of the principal but uniquely identifies the trainee by means of a suffix.

A dentist may be exempt from the requirement to complete vocational training if his or her name has been included in a dental list in the UK within the period of five years ending on the date of the application to be included in the dental list or he or she has practised in primary dental care for a period of at least four years in aggregate in either the Community Dental Service or the armed forces.

Associates

An associate agreement as defined in the NHS regulations is:

> ... an agreement between dentists practising as principals –

(a) to which there are two parties, not being partners of each other,
(b) whereby one party is liable to provide, for financial consideration, the use of some or all premises and of some or all facilities for the provision of general dental services.

The dentist who provides the premises and/or facilities is known as the first party associate. The dentist making use of the premises/facilities provided is known as the second party associate.

Principal

A principal is the dentist who takes responsibility for the services provided under a contract. A dentist may be a principal in one or more contracts at any time. It is for the dentist to decide how many contracts he or she has and how they are used.

The dentist who holds a contract as a principal at one address may also be an assistant or associate at other addresses but not at the same address.

Contract numbers

Each contract is identified by a unique 14-digit contract number issued by the DPB. The contract number is made up of four parts.

- Digits 1–3 indicate the health authority (GDS) or pilot number (PDS).
- Digits 4–9 make up the dentist's personal number. It uniquely identifies the dentist and is issued by the DPB once the dentist has initially

registered with the General Dental Council and stays with the dentist for the whole time he or she practises in the NHS.

- Digits 10–12 are for a partnership which again is a unique number. Most contracts are not percentage-sharing partnerships and so will show /000/ as a partnership number.
- Digits 13 and 14 are the suffix number which identifies something special about the contract, e.g. assistants have a suffix number 81–89, and are also issued by the DPB.

The Regulations

The obligations and responsibilities that dentists must assume when practising in the NHS are contained in the NHS (General Dental Services) Regulations 1992 (as amended), known as 'the Regulations'.

This piece of secondary legislation, Statutory Instrument 1992 No. 661, was made by the Secretary of State for Health using powers conferred on him by the National Health Service Act 1977 (as amended). A copy of the document is provided to each dentist when he or she begins to provide dental services within the NHS. It is not necessary to look at the Regulations in fine detail. Below are those areas considered to be of particular relevance for a dentist entering the NHS GDS for the first time.

The interpretation section is to be found in Part I and defines the more common terms in daily usage; for example, 'care and treatment' means:

(a) all proper and necessary care which a dentist usually undertakes for a patient and which the patient is willing to undergo, including advice, planning of treatment and preventive care, and
(b) treatment;

'Treatment' is defined separately and includes:

examination, diagnosis, preventive treatment, periodontal treatment, conservative treatment, surgical treatment, the supply and repair of dental appliances, orthodontic treatment and the taking of radiographs and the provision of general anaesthesia and sedation in connection with such treatment and the supply of listed drugs and the issue of prescriptions . . .

'Care and treatment' is the cornerstone of everything dentists provide for their patients.

Part III of the Regulations sets out the 'General arrangements for provision of general dental services'. This part of the Regulations is important as it gives details about the dental list prepared by each health authority; how to apply to be included in such a dental list; removal and withdrawal from the dental list and health authority arrangements for the provision of emergency cover.

Part IV deals with the 'Remuneration of dentists' and considers not only the approval of payments made to dentists but also the method by which an overpayment may be recovered.

However, probably the most important part of the Regulations is Schedule 1 where the Terms of Service for dentists are set out in detail. The detail of the Terms of Service is not given here but all dentists working within the NHS should familiarise themselves with Schedule 1 and have the document available for reference when in doubt.

We will now consider the more common breaches of the Terms of Service but before doing so, it must be stated that the vast majority of dentists go through the whole of their careers without contravening the Regulations.

Standards of care (paragraph 20(1)(a) & 20(1)(d))

The Regulations state that: 'In providing general dental services, a dentist shall employ a proper degree of skill and attention'. The term is mandatory and concerns:

- diagnosis
- treatment planning
- provision of treatment

so that the oral health of the patient is secured and maintained.

Failure to secure the oral health of the patient, except in the case of occasional treatment and when providing treatment on referral, through poor diagnosis, treatment planning and provision of treatment is considered a failure to 'employ a proper degree of skill and attention'.

Unnecessary treatment (paragraph 20(c))

'... a dentist shall not provide care and treatment in excess of that which is necessary to secure and maintain oral health'. Again the requirement is mandatory and it goes without saying that if it is established that excessive treatment is either proposed or is actually provided, then the dentist is considered to be in breach of this regulation.

Claiming appropriately (paragraph 19(1)(a) & (b))

Unless the Regulations provide otherwise:

> A dentist shall not claim or accept the payment of any fee or other remuneration in respect of any treatment –
>
> (a) which he has provided under the general dental services; or
> (b) which has not been provided or for which another claim has already been submitted . . . for payment.

A dentist therefore must only claim fees from the NHS in accordance with the narrative contained in the Statement of Dental Remuneration:

- for work that has actually been done and
- for work which has not been claimed for already.

Mixing NHS and private treatment

An area that causes much confusion is that of 'mixing' NHS and private treatment for a patient on the same course of treatment. Paragraphs 4 and 5 refer to continuing care and capitation arrangements respectively. Paragraph 16 refers to the mixing of NHS treatment and private care and treatment.

Where there is to be a 'mixing' of NHS and private treatment for patients registered under either a continuing care or a capitation arrangement, the dentist must make sure that:

- patients must give consent to the proposed private treatment
- patients must not be advised that treatment necessary under a continuing care arrangement is not available under the NHS GDS
- patients must not be misled about the quality and care of treatment available under the NHS GDS
- if treatment necessary to secure oral health relates to a single tooth, treatment shall be wholly under the NHS GDS or wholly private.

Records

The keeping of satisfactory records is of paramount importance and cannot be stressed too often. Well-documented records are vitally important and particularly so in circumstances when allegations of any kind are made against a dentist. The patient's records will form the basis of the defence to any such allegations. Record cards (FP25/25a) are provided for use in the general dental services.

- The standard of record keeping is covered in paragraph 25(1).
- There is a requirement to retain the records for two years after completion of a course of treatment (paragraph 25(2)).
- A further requirement is that, if requested, a dentist will submit a patient's records to the authority, the Dental Practice Board or a Dental Reference Officer within 14 days of being required to do so.

Prior approval (paragraph 26(1)(a) & (b))

A dentist must submit to the Dental Practice Board without unreasonable delay an estimate of the whole care and treatment, including details of any private treatment:

- when the total amount of NHS fees according to the Statement of Dental Remuneration is above £230, or
- where, according to the Statement of Dental Remuneration, any item of treatment requires prior approval of the Dental Practice Board.

A dentist, except in an emergency, must not proceed with any treatment until he receives prior approval from the Dental Practice Board. Dentists who persistently fail to observe the rule concerning prior approval applications may find themselves not only in trouble but also out of pocket when payment is refused.

The role of the Dental Practice Board

The Dental Practice Board (DPB) is a statutory body set up originally under the National Health Service Act 1946 and now under the National Health Service Act 1977 as amended by the Health and Medicines Act 1988. The DPB is centrally financed and sponsored by the Department of Health.

As such, it is accountable to the Secretary of State for Health and the National Assembly for Wales.

The principal functions of the DPB are:

- approval of payment applications
- calculating and transferring payments
- preventing and detecting fraud and abuse
- providing dental health information.

At the time of writing there are about 17 000 dentists working in the GDS as principals providing NHS treatment. Patients are required to pay a statutory charge of 80% towards the cost of any one course of treatment up to a maximum amount, currently £348. The dentist is responsible for collecting the patients' charges; the balance of the fees due to the dentist is paid by the DPB. Certain groups of patients are exempt from patient charges irrespective of their ability to pay. These include patients under 18, those who are over 18 but who are in full-time education, expectant mothers and nursing mothers. Those who are on low incomes may be exempt from paying the charges either in full or in part, depending on the particular circumstances.

The government has been concerned about the availability of and access to dental treatment in certain geographical areas of England and Wales. In an effort to improve matters, health authorities in such areas have been encouraged to pilot schemes aimed at raising the level of oral health.

The 1997 NHS (Primary Care) Act introduced the concept of Personal Dental Services (PDS). The Act required patients to pay the same charge in the PDS as they would pay in the GDS. The initial PDS schemes covered a wide variation of treatment 'providers', ranging from dental hygienists and therapists working under the direction of a dentist to dentists providing specialist treatments such as orthodontics, oral surgery or anaesthetics.

It was, therefore, inevitable that the DPB would become intimately involved with these new initiatives in the organisation and provision of payment and probity systems for the schemes. PDS payment arrangements depend on the type of scheme involved. They include the usual item-of-service payments but also payments for block contracts, performance thresholds, salaries and sessional fees. The whole concept of PDS provided an enormous task for the DPB to undertake and the organisation responded effectively to the challenge.

Dentists working in the GDS receive payment in accordance with the schedule of authorised fees detailed in the Statement of Dental Remuneration (SDR). The SDR sets out the current scale of fees for work carried out in the GDS. The fees are itemised according to the type of treatment and each item is given a code number. The SDR indicates the gross fee that a dentist may claim and the corresponding patient charge for the particular item of treatment. The gross fees include amounts for practice expenses, laboratory charges and time spent at the chairside. Some fees for 'special' items of treatment are at the discretion of the DPB and may require prior approval. It must be stressed that only authorised fees contained in the SDR are allowed under the GDS. Guides produced by other organisations may be helpful for quick and easy reference but should not be relied upon for their content. If dentists are in doubt about entitlement to a fee or the correct fee to claim, then they must consult the current edition of the SDR. No other source of information should be regarded as authoritative or reliable.

The primary function of the DPB is to pay dentists promptly and accurately. Each dentist holding a contract number and providing services in the GDS receives a payment schedule every month from the DPB. In the year to the end of March 1999, the DPB paid 99.1% of claims for payment on the first month after the claim was submitted, 99.9% of which were correct.

Assurance in the GDS

A further important role of the DPB is to assure the government and the taxpayer that the GDS is providing a quality service which is cost effective. The DPB provides the evidence through its monitoring and probity functions. Four distinct areas of GDS activity come under DPB scrutiny:

- the quality of diagnosis and treatment planning
- quality of treatment provided
- the compliance of dentists with their Terms of Service
- the accuracy of claims submitted for payment.

The probity checks carried out by the DPB fall into two categories: random or screening checks on a dentist's activity and specific or targeted checks made on activity which appears to be anomalous. Only those dentists registered with the General Dental Council are allowed to practise in the GDS. The DPB believes that such registered dentists are honest and willing to abide by the GDS regulations. This supposition enables the DPB to carry out post-payment rather than pre-payment checks whilst maintaining the prompt payment code demanded by government.

A series of validation checks are made to ensure that dentists receive payment only in accordance with the SDR. DPB screening checks may be statistical, administrative or clinical. Approximately 34 million applications for payment are made each year and they provide an enormous amount of statistical data whereby patterns of activity and anomalies can be identified. Administrative screening is carried out through inspection of patients' records and supporting radiographs. Questionnaires are used to seek the patient's recollection of events surrounding a particular course of treatment. However, such an administrative procedure does not provide evidence of the need for and quality of treatment carried out. This can only be provided through clinical examination.

The Dental Reference Service

The Dental Reference Service (DRS) is part of the DPB. It consists of approximately 60 Dental Reference Officers (DRO) divided into six teams covering the whole of England and Wales. A DRO undergoes a period of training on appointment and many have special knowledge and skills. All DROs have considerable experience of working in the GDS. The DPB is committed to the ongoing training of its DROs through regular update courses and through calibration. In this way DROs are kept fully abreast of current clinical thinking and techniques. Regular calibration ensures that a high degree of consistency between DROs is achieved.

The DRS, through its DROs, carries out about 84 000 clinical examinations per year of patients who have received treatment in the GDS or PDS. These examinations form a vital part in the process by which government and public are assured that diagnosis and the provision of treatment in the GDS and PDS are of a high standard.

In the year to the end of March 1999, fewer than 1.5% of DRO examinations revealed a serious concern about the diagnosis or treatment provided.

The DRO reports on each examination carried out and gives the report a particular code. All adversely coded reports are scrutinised by a Senior Dental Officer and forwarded for further probity checks. Dentists receiving an adversely coded report may be asked for their comments or observations. They may be asked to submit the patient's records and radiographs. In serious cases the file may be passed to the DPB Reference Committee for consideration regarding possible breaches of the Terms of Service. The Reference Committee consists of the Head of Information and Probity, a Dental Adviser and a Senior Dental Officer.

The Committee may decide:

- to refer the case to the appropriate health authority for consideration; in this case the matter is ratified by the Chief Dental Adviser

- to issue a warning letter to the dentist
- to issue a letter of concern
- that some other form of action is appropriate.

It is often forgotten that another important role of the DPB is to provide statistical information for the health authorities of England and Wales. Dental Data Services are a division of the DPB that produces a wide range of publications on GDS statistics. Data are available in published form and on 3.5″ computer disk. The DPB welcomes enquiries from interested parties and is happy to discuss the provision of data in specified formats. In this role the DPB can help health authorities to carry out research projects. Contact Dental Data Services on 01323 433218.

Finally, the DPB Helpdesk is there to answer questions from dentists and patients alike (01323 433550).

NHS complaints and disciplinary procedures

Growing dissatisfaction from professionals and patients resulted in the government setting up a complete review of NHS complaints procedures in the early 1990s under the chairmanship of Professor Wilson (Leeds University). The ensuing report concluded that new arrangements for dealing with complaints were urgently required. The new arrangements were introduced in April 1996. The main difference from the 'old' system is the separation of complaints and disciplinary matters.

Complaints

This procedure has been put in place to resolve disputes between dentists and patients.

Each practice must have a complaints procedure with one person delegated the responsibility for its administration. The practice procedure should be publicised to the patients and it is a requirement that records are kept of any complaint handled within the practice. The process is known as local resolution. The record of the complaint should be kept separate from the patient's clinical records.

All complaints should be acknowledged in writing within two working days and following investigation of the complaint, a written response should be sent to the patient within 10 working days of the original complaint. If the patient is not satisfied with the outcome, he/she can ask the local health authority/health board (HA/HB) to look at the matter.

Each HA/HB has a convenor who will look at the case and decide on the next course of action. This can include:

- referring the complaint back to the practice
- conciliation
- independent review
- advising the patient of his/her right to contact the Health Services Ombudsman
- no further action.

If the HA/HB convenor decides to set up an independent review panel, the panel will be assisted in clinical matters by qualified dentists from a list nominated by the Local Dental Committee. A copy of the panel's report is sent to the two parties and the HA/HB for it to decide whether or not further action is necessary. Further action may be of a disciplinary nature.

Disciplinary action

This procedure deals with possible breaches of a dentist's Terms of Service under the GDS Regulations.

Disciplinary action is taken by the HA/HB on whose list the dentist is included. The HA/HB may receive information about possible breaches of Terms of Service in a number of ways, including:

- written patient complaint
- Dental Reference Officer report
- information from the Dental Practice Board.

A subcommittee of the HA/HB, the Reference Committee, decides if any action is to be taken. The Reference Committee has access to clinical advice. Possible courses of action are:

- no further action
- to refer the matter to:

  - a Dental Disciplinary Committee (DDC)
  - an NHS tribunal

- the General Dental Council
- the police
- a combination of the above.

If the HA/HB decides to refer the matter to a DDC the matter is dealt with by another HA/HB who, provided the referral has been made within the strict time limits specified within the GDS Regulations, must convene their DDC.

The referring HA/HB must within 28 days of the referral send a Statement of Case to the dentist and the DDC. The dentist has 28 days from the date it is sent to respond to the Statement of Case. Twenty-one days' notice must be given of the date, time and place of the hearing to all interested parties.

The DDC has a legally qualified chairman and either two or three dental members and either two or three lay members. There must be an equal number of dental and lay members hearing the case. Both parties may be represented by another person at the hearing. However, the person presenting the case must not be legally qualified. The dentist is usually represented by his or her defence organisation. There is no set procedure for the hearing and evidence is not taken on oath. Both parties and their witnesses may give evidence and can be cross-examined by the other party and by members of the committee. If a patient is involved he or she is usually examined by the dental members of the committee. The dentist may also examine the patient. When all the evidence has been heard, the committee makes its decision. The deliberations are held in private. The decision of the committee is taken on the civil standard of proof, i.e. on the balance of probability. The DDC reports to the referring HA/HB, setting out its recommendations for any further action. The referring HA/HB must accept the report's findings but may alter the recommendations of further action.

Recommendations that a DDC may make include:

- no further action
- warn the dentist to comply more closely with his/her Terms of Service
- witholding a sum of money from the dentist's remuneration
- a period of prior approval.

The dentist has the right of appeal against the decision of the HA/HB. Any appeal must be lodged within 30 days of him/her receiving the decision. The appeal is made to the HA/HB who may decide to hold an oral hearing of appeal. The panel appointed to hear the appeal comprises a legally qualified chairman, a dentist selected from members of the General Dental Services Committee of the British Dental Association and a Dental Officer of the Department of Health. Evidence is taken on oath and the parties may be legally represented. In Scotland the right of appeal is to the Secretary of State.

NHS tribunal

A dentist may be called to appear before an NHS tribunal for persistent serious breaches of the GDS Regulations. In such cases the HA/HB will apply for a hearing before the tribunal. The NHS tribunal consists of a chairman appointed by the Lord Chancellor together with one dental member and one lay member appointed by the Secretary of State. Evidence is taken on oath. The tribunal has only one sanction it can impose which is to debar the dentist from inclusion on the list of any or all HAs/HBs and subsequently from practice within the GDS.

The Health Service Commissioner for England, Wales and Scotland

Otherwise known as the Health Service Ombudsman. The word 'Ombudsman' is of Scandinavian origin and literally means 'Freedom's man'.

The Parliamentary Commissioner for Administration (Ombudsman) was established in Britain in 1967 to examine complaints of maladministration. However, it was not until 1973 that the Health Service Commissioner came into being. The three Health Service Ombudsman posts, and that of Parliamentary Ombudsman, have so far always been held by the same person. The appointment is made by the Crown and is currently held by Michael Buckley. Apart from the appointment, the powers and jurisdiction of the Ombudsman are governed by the Health Service Commissioners Act 1993 (as amended).

The Ombudsman is completely independent of government and the NHS but is accountable to Parliament.

The Health Service Commissioners (Amendment) Act 1996 gave the Ombudsman the power to investigate complaints about services provided by those working in the NHS, from health authorities and healthcare trusts to individual primary care providers such as doctors and dentists. The new powers came into force on 1 April 1996 and are not retrospective.

Certain types of complaint are outside the Ombudsman's jurisdiction. These include complaints about:

- personnel issues such as appointments of staff, pay or discipline
- the disciplinary procedures introduced in 1996 that replaced the old service committees
- matters where the person making the complaint can pursue an action and obtain a remedy through the courts, e.g. where there is a claim for

damages arising through professional negligence or a right of appeal or review before a tribunal. The General Dental Council is not regarded as a tribunal for this purpose.

There is a one-year time limit imposed on complainants to bring their complaint after which the Ombudsman cannot investigate a complaint unless he considers it is reasonable to waive that limit in the interests of justice. It is complaints about clinical judgement that relate to the patient's treatment or care that are of concern to the practising dentist. The majority of complaints to the Ombudsman concern independent reviews under the new NHS complaints procedures which have gone against the complainant or cases in which there has been a refusal to hold an independent review.

The Ombudsman requires professional help in cases involving clinical matters and a Dental Adviser to the Ombudsman has been appointed on a part-time basis.

When a complaint arrives at the Ombudsman's office, a file is opened and much information is collected, including statements from the complainant, the dentist complained of, any hospitals to which the patient was referred, health authorities and any other party involved in the case.

At this stage the Dental Adviser reads the file and weighs up the evidence to assess whether there is merit in a full investigation. The Dental Adviser's decision to proceed is made if there appears to have been some injustice and an investigation would be beneficial to resolve the matter. The final decision on whether or not to proceed to a full investigation is not taken by the Dental Adviser. He or she advises the Commission who makes the decision.

About 10% of complaints referred to the Ombudsman go on to a full investigation. If a case is investigated then the Dental Adviser will appoint two External Professional Advisers (EPA) from a list provided by the Department of Health and approved by the British Dental Association. The EPAs appointed will usually be of a similar age, qualification and experience to the dentists complained of. Confidentiality is maintained and the EPAs do not know the identity of the dentist complained of.

The EPAs act, in effect, as peer judges. Using their own knowledge, experience and expertise, they take account of the skills, knowledge and experience of the dentist concerned. The EPAs will decide whether the dentist's action were based on a reasonable and responsible exercise of clinical judgement in the circumstances, taking into account the standard of good clinical practice. In reaching their conclusions the EPAs use the civil law test of the balance of probabilities.

So, in practical terms, the EPAs meet with the Dental Adviser to decide how the case will be investigated. This usually involves study of the case notes, relevant radiographs, letters, interviews with the dentist, complainant, staff and sometimes consultants to whom the case has been referred, and any other witnesses. The EPAs write a joint report advising the Ombudsman of their findings and conclusion. The EPAs therefore decide whether what the dentist did was reasonable in the circumstances. This draft report is sent to all parties for agreement.

The final report of any investigation is the sole responsibility of the Ombudsman who has a responsibility to be wholly objective, impartial and transparent. The Ombudsman seeks to be fair to all the parties concerned.

The Health Service Commissioners Act 1993 gives absolute privilege and freedom from any action in defamation in respect of any final report published by the Ombudsman. The Ombudsman and members of his staff cannot be called to give evidence in legal proceedings arising out of an investigation.

The legislation extends the powers of the Ombudsman so that he can disclose information, discovered during the course of an investigation which would otherwise be protected by the rules of confidentiality, to a statutory regulatory body such as the General Dental Council.

It should be said that what the majority of complainants want most of all is to be given honest answers in terms they can understand from open, impartial enquiries. Though the powers of the Ombudsman are considerable the need to resort to those powers ought to arise only in exceptional circumstances.

Acknowledgements

I wish to thank the following for their help and assistance in putting together this chapter: Sam Barsam (former Senior Dental Adviser at the Dental Practice Board) for writing the opening remarks; Elaine Pearson (Dental Contracts Manager at the Dental Practice Board) for her help in providing the material on dental contracts; Martin Wall (Dental Reference Officer, Dental Practice Board, and former member of North Yorkshire Local Dental Committee) for writing the section on NHS complaint and discipline procedures; and Mervyn Yewe-Dyer (Dental Adviser to the Ombudsman) for supplying the information used in the section on the Ombudsman.

Further reading

- *The National Health Service (General Dental Services) Regulations 1992* (as amended).
- Dental Practice Board (1999) *Annual Review 1998–99*.
- *A Guide to the Work of the Health Service Ombudsman*.
- Beveridge W (1942) *Social Insurance and Allied Services*. HMSO, London.

- Harris J (1997) *William Beveridge: a biography.* Oxford University Press, Oxford.
- Hollander S (1978) *The Economics of John Stuart Mill. Volume 2.* Open University Press, Buckingham.
- Ranade W (1997) *A Future for the NHS?* Longmans, Harlow.
- Webster C (1998) *The National Health Service: a political history.* Oxford University Press, Oxford.

CHAPTER TWELVE

Negligence and litigation

Greg Waldron

It is often said that complaints are the precursors of litigation. A complaint, in whatever form it arises, provides an opportunity for resolution but if it is not resolved, the patient may resort to litigation. The law regarding professional negligence, and the usual legal process, is often complex and this chapter can only therefore be seen as an outline and overview of litigation in England and Wales.

Negligence

To succeed in a dental claim a patient ('claimant') has the burden of proof which means that they must show that the dentist was negligent. The three essentials that claimants must prove in every case are:

- duty of care and breach of that duty
- causation
- harm/injury.

Unless all three 'essential ingredients' are present, the claim will not succeed.

Duty of care and breach (liability)

It is well established that a dentist owes a duty of care to patients and that duty is not to harm or injure them. Any injury can occur by an action or an omission (failure to act). If a dentist injures a patient as a result of incorrect treatment, then the duty of care may have been breached if the dentist has not provided treatment to the acceptable clinical standard. To establish whether a dentist has breached the duty of care it is therefore essential to initially investigate whether the treatment provided was of the applicable standard. It should also be noted that dentists are also responsible for the actions of their employees (assistant dentists, nurses and receptionists), if the negligent act is performed in the course of their employment, under the doctrine of vicarious liability.[1]

Standard of care

The fundamental test for breach of duty in the tort of negligence is whether the conduct was reasonable in all the circumstances of the case. The legal test of professional breach of duty is established as the Bolam test[2] and this has been widely considered in subsequent clinical negligence cases. Dentists are to be judged by whether they have reached the standard of:

> the ordinarily skilled man exercising or professing to have that special skill. A man need not possess the highest expert skill at the risk of being found negligent ... it is sufficient if he exercises the ordinary skill of an ordinary competent man exercising that particular art.[3]

Therefore if a dentist carries out a complicated clinical procedure for the first time ever, such as an implant, the dentist would have to demonstrate that he or she exercised the augmented skill of a dentist experienced in that particular clinical procedure rather than the ordinary skill of a general dental practitioner. It is established that to claim clinical inexperience is no defence and so an 'incompetent best' will not be good enough.[4] In considering breach of duty a dentist's education, experience, training and the currency of knowledge may be closely examined. Importantly, the nature of dental knowledge and practice at the time of the clinical event in question is to be taken into account when considering the applicable standard of care.[5]

Evidence of the skill the dentist should have applied is provided by appropriate experts and, for example, in general dental practice cases an experienced general dental practitioner would be instructed to give an opinion as to whether the dentist complied with the applicable standard. The law accepts that there may be differing bodies of professional opinion and practice and that a dentist would not be negligent if he or she acted 'in accordance with such a practice, merely because there is a body of opinion that takes a contrary view'.[2] So, if a dentist can demonstrate that a reasonable body of professional opinion would have treated the patient in the same way then that will successfully defend a claim but only as long as the body of professional opinion is seen to be reasonable, responsible and logical. A judge may possibly find that the professional opinion defending the dentist is unreasonable, irresponsible and illogical[6] and so, despite the dentist having carried out a procedure in common usage, find that the dentist has breached the duty of care. If a claimant can show that the dentist's treatment failed to reach the accepted standard then the next stage is to consider causation.

Breach of contract

If treatment has been provided privately then patients can also sue for breach of contract if the treatment is not successful or not performed in accordance with the agreement. More importantly, the claimant does not have to show that the dentist was negligent but only that the treatment provided was not of the required standard to succeed. The treatment provided must be of 'satisfactory' quality[7] and the test is the quality that would be acceptable to a reasonable patient. Treatment must be fit for the purpose, free from minor defects, of good appearance, safe and durable in order to be of satisfactory quality. If the treatment in question is not found to be of satisfactory quality then the patient is entitled to reject it and is also entitled to compensation for any injury, or harm, that may flow (see below) just as if the dentist had been negligent.

Causation

Whereas the test in criminal cases is 'beyond reasonable doubt' (i.e. almost certain) in civil claims the test is 'the balance of probabilities' (i.e. more likely than not).[8] The claimant must therefore show that the injury suffered, despite other possible causes, was more likely than not caused by the dentist's action or omission. In simpler terms if expert opinion is that, on a percentage basis, the dentist's act or omission was probably 51% or more likely to be the cause of the injury and another, possibly natural, cause was 49% or less, then the claimant will succeed in establishing causation.

Harm/injury

Claimants must then demonstrate the injury they have suffered. It is established that mere distress cannot be claimed for, although it is possible to claim for a recognised psychological injury, such as post-traumatic stress disorder.[9] The claimant must be able to show actual physical injury and will need to bring expert evidence to support the nature of the injuries.

So, if a claimant can show that the dentist breached the duty of care in the treatment and on a balance of probabilities it caused injury, he or she is then able to move on to consider the entitlement to compensation.

Compensation

The only remedy for injury in civil claims is money. Claimants are usually awarded 'general' and 'special' damages. Compensation is usually paid in dental cases on a 'once-and-for-all' settlement and provisional damages (further payment if a possible future event occurs) settlements are rare.

It should be noted that a claimant is under a duty to 'mitigate their loss'. It can take some considerable time for a case to come to trial, or be settled, after an injury and claimants should obtain timely and appropriate corrective treatment for their injury and so not extend their suffering, or the seriousness of the injury, by waiting until the outcome of a trial, or settlement, before receiving such treatment. Where a claimant refuses treatment which could have lessened the consequences of the injury, the claimant must show that his/her refusal was reasonable.[10]

General damages

General damages are an award for the pain and suffering associated with the injury suffered. The amount is calculated with reference to previous judgements in cases regarding similar injuries or guidelines.[11] If the relevant case is many years old then the amount of general damages is calculated to the present day value using the Retail Prices Index.

Special damages

Special damages are an award of damages specific to the claimant's injury and the individual circumstances that flow from their injury. In dental claims common special damages claims are for treatment costs, travelling expenses in attending for treatment, prescription charges, loss of earnings, etc. The major special damages claim is usually for the costs of corrective treatment and, if applicable, future replacement treatment costs.

It is a fundamental legal principle that claimants are entitled to be placed in the position they would have been but for the negligence. Therefore if, for example, they have lost a tooth, they are entitled to have a replacement tooth provided by a clinically feasible method which may be an implant, bridge or a denture. Additionally, if the recommended treatment needs replacing at regular intervals then they will be entitled to claim all future replacement costs over their expected lifetime as long as the particular treatment required is a new procedure (i.e. not a straightforward replacement) which they wouldn't have needed but for the negligence. Starting with the present-day cost of treatment, the expected replacement cycle period and the claimant's likely life expectancy, a complicated actuarial calculation is performed to arrive at a lump sum which, if invested, would provide for the expected treatment costs over the claimant's lifetime.

It is also established that claimants are entitled to claim the costs of private corrective treatment over their lifetime despite the fact that it may have been NHS treatment that failed.

Aggravated damages

Aggravated damages may be awarded if a dentist's conduct was found to have injured the claimant's feelings of dignity and pride. Such awards are very rare but have been made in a leading dental case[12] where a dentist was found to have committed a battery by carrying out unnecessary work and so the claimants recovered for general damages at an enhanced rate to reflect this.

Interest

Claimants are also entitled to claim interest on damages which is calculated from the date of the clinical event giving rise to the claim.

Increasing levels of damages

The value of dental claims generally seems to be increasing and this may well be due to the more sophisticated corrective treatments, and particularly implants, that are now widely available to patients.

Compensation recovery

If a claimant has claimed certain state benefits as a result of the alleged injury then, if the case is successful, the benefits paid will be effectively deducted from any eventual compensation by the Compensation Recovery Unit. This type of recovery rarely occurs in dental cases as claimants generally do not usually find themselves unable to work, or greatly disabled, as a result of the injury. It is also worth noting that if a claimant on state benefits is paid considerable compensation, that is, more than the upper limit on capital for certain means-tested benefits, this can, perhaps unfairly, stop them receiving that state benefit until their means dwindle. If claimants may face such a dilemma then they can circumvent the problem by placing the compensation in a special needs trust fund where they are the only beneficiary.

The legal process

If a patient sues they will generally use a solicitor who specialises in clinical negligence cases. Some patients attempt to bring a case by themselves and are known as 'litigants in person'. The same rules apply to litigants in person although they often are inexperienced in the court rules and this can cause confusion to all involved in the legal process. This account will only consider the usual position where a patient has instructed a solicitor and how such a claim will be dealt with.

Legal costs

The fundamental position is that the loser in a case pays the winner's legal costs in addition to his or her own. If a claimant discontinues the case once court proceedings have been issued then he/she is also responsible for his/her opponent's costs. It is only when a claimant is legally aided that he or she is not generally responsible for the dentist's costs if unsuccessful. Legal costs can be substantial due to the often technically complicated nature of dental negligence cases and generally costs are greater than the amount of compensation paid. Legal costs will also be paid if a case is settled at any stage.

All dentists must be indemnified against negligence claims.[13] Dentists will be assisted and should be represented by their defence organisation in any claim that will deal with all correspondence so that the dentist is not directly contacted by the claimant's solicitors. The dentist's defence organisation should pay all the applicable legal costs along with any compensation which is subsequently due.

Claimant funding

As soon as a claimant goes to a solicitor he or she must consider how to fund the pursuit of the claim. Some claimants may still be eligible for Legal Aid, now called public funding, although its availability is becoming greatly restricted. An increasing number of claimants are funding claims backed by legal expenses insurance that they have as part of their household buildings and contents policy. With both Legal Aid and legal expenses insurance, claimants are at no risk of paying legal costs if the case is lost and so it could be said that they have little to risk in bringing a claim. A small number of claimants fund claims privately but the threat of paying the legal costs if the case is lost can be a deterrent to proceeding.

There has also been a rise in the number of cases being progressed on conditional ('no win, no fee') fee agreements backed by an expensive insurance policy to pay legal costs if the case is lost. An additional success fee is paid to the claimant's solicitor if the case is won. The court can order the success fee and insurance premium to be paid as additional legal costs if the claimant wins the case.[14] Present conditional fee agreements have made litigation more accessible and therefore may prove to be an attractive option for claimants. The government's continuing restrictions on Legal Aid should make the use of this method of funding more prevalent.

Claimant – initial investigation

The claimant's solicitor will need to initially investigate the merits of the claimant's case. The starting point will be for the solicitor to request copies of the records from the dentist. These must be provided to the claimant's solicitor within 40 days and standard fees can be charged for providing copies.[15] The dentist should immediately contact his or her defence organisation at this stage who will assist in dealing with this request. The fact that copy records have been requested is no guarantee that a claim will definitely ensue but should put the dentist on notice of a possibility of a claim. Once the solicitors have obtained the records then they will investigate the case and frequently they will obtain an initial expert report in order to decide whether the case is of merit. This initial report has great significance to the funding arrangements of cases for if the initial report is not supportive then the Legal Aid Board, or any prospective insurer, will not fund the case. If the expert's report is positive then the case may proceed to the next stage of sending a letter of claim.

Multiple dentists/claimants

It may be that the events in question cover a long period of time and a number of dentists. It is therefore not unusual for a claimant to sue a number of dentists in one claim as they may be jointly and severally liable. If a claimant can show that a dentist was at least in part to blame (even as low as 1%) out of a number of dentists then he/she is entitled to recover all the damages, and costs, against that one dentist. If a number of dentists are sued in one case and they belong to different defence organisations, then the different defence organisations will usually agree on which one should take the lead in defending the claim and ultimately apportion between them the payment of any damages. This makes the litigation process more manageable.

There have been cases where a number of claimants have pursued one dentist with similar claims.[12] These cases are not perhaps genuine 'multi-party cases' because each claimant has not experienced the same event. The individual claimants may have been treated by the same dentist, at the same place, in the same period and in a similar manner as the other claimants and so it is logical to consolidate the cases at one court hearing for ease of management and also to ensure a consistency of approach. This does not in any way prevent the court from considering each individual claim on its own facts and merits.

Dentist's initial investigation

The request for records will usually mean that the dentist's defence organisation will initially consider the potential claim. Due to tight legal deadlines there is considerable pressure to investigate cases at an early stage as any delay may later result in court-administered penalties. With this in mind, if it appears that the claim may have some validity a full investigation may be commenced at this stage rather than waiting for the claimant's solicitor to produce a letter of claim.

Letter of claim and offer to settle

This letter is intended to set out fully the claimant's case. It must comply with court directions[16] and contain a clear summary of the facts, the main allegations of negligence and the causal link with injuries, details of the claimant's injuries and condition and prognosis and details of financial losses. The court's clear intention is that at this stage the dentist should understand fully the case to be answered and the defence organisation should be able to calculate the likely value of the claim. The claimant's case must also only deal with relevant issues that are proportionate to the value of the case in accordance with the over-riding rules of litigation.[17] The dentist will be interviewed in order to obtain recollections, discuss potential implications and to decide how to deal with the claim (if this investigation has not already been attended to in response to the request for records). The defence organisation may also at this stage obtain initial expert opinion in order to help consider whether the claim may be valid or defensible and, further, whether settlement should be negotiated. The claimant must give the dentist and the defence organisation 90 days to consider and respond to the letter of claim before issuing proceedings unless there should be a 'limitation' problem (see below).

The claimant may, if they wish, include an 'offer to settle'[18] which sets out the amount he/she would accept to settle the claim. The offer is deemed to be open for 21 days and may have important future costs consequences if not accepted. If eventually the case is settled for the same amount or less, then the Court would take the view that the offer should have been accepted early on and penalty will be made when assessing legal costs at the conclusion of the case.

Dentist's response

The dentist and his or her defence organisation have 90 days to consider the letter of claim and must respond fully to all the issues within this period. The court's rationale is that at the end of this process the issues in most cases should be clear and hopefully resolution may occur without resort to costly, time-consuming and stressful litigation. The letter may also include an offer to settle on behalf of the dentist that can likewise have costs consequences for the claimant if the same or a lesser amount is ultimately accepted.

Experts

The basis of the Bolam test is very much akin to the concept of 'peer review/ audit'. Both sides will generally provide expert opinion although the court has the power to instruct both parties to use a single joint expert.[19] The expert instructed must report within his or her own area of expertise and also comply with detailed court directions.[20] Often a number of different experts may report in one case. For example, in a periodontal claim arising out of general dental practice an experienced general dental practitioner will be required to report into breach of duty, a periodontal expert to report regarding causation and a restorative expert to report on corrective and future treatment needs. The implications of using a large number of experts for the complexity and costs of such litigation should be readily apparent.

Court proceedings

The claim form

If the case has not been resolved at the pre-action protocol stage then the claimant must consider whether or not to issue court proceedings. The letter of response may make it clear that the dentist's defence organisation considers that there is no case to answer. If the claimant decides to proceed then he or she will have to issue a 'claim form'. This is an official court document that sets out the claimant's case in more detail than the letter of claim. The claim form must have attached to it an expert report substantiating the injuries and a schedule detailing all the special damages claims. Once the claim form is issued at a court it must be served on the dentist within four months. The dentist is now properly referred to as 'the defendant'.

Limitation

Generally the law on limitation is that claimants must issue proceedings before the third anniversary of the date on which they became aware they had suffered an injury or they are 'time barred' from doing so. If the date of injury is clear there is no problem in applying this rule and if otherwise, the law on limitation is somewhat complex[21] and beyond the scope of this chapter. It is common in dental claims for claimants only to become potentially aware that they have suffered harm when they change dentists. Upon investigation of their claim it may become clear that the clinical event that caused the injury may have taken place more than three years before they changed dentists and subsequently first considered the possibility of negligence. On a strict interpretation of the 'three year rule' they would be barred from bringing a claim but it will most probably be interpreted that the three years run from the date on which the new dentist informed them of a potential problem and, in such circumstances, the court would probably use its discretion[22] to allow the case to proceed.

The defence

Once the claim form has been served then the dentist has up to 28 days in which to serve a defence which must fully address all the allegations and issues contained in the claim form. Once the defence is served then the court will provide both parties with an allocation questionnaire which requires detailed information of the number of witnesses and experts the parties may call, in which court track the parties wish the case to be heard and whether the parties would like a stay of the proceedings for a month in order to see whether they can settle the case. Once the allocation question-naire is returned to the court it will be looked at by a judge, along with the claim form and defence, who will then decide how to manage the case.[23]

The court track

There are three potential court tracks that may be followed. Small claims for simple claims under £5000, the fast track for claims less than £15 000 in value which are suitable for a one-day hearing and the multi-track for all other cases. The multi-track is likely to be the preferred track for dental negligence cases and it is most likely that the judge will then schedule an initial case management conference to decide the timetable up to trial. Depending upon the value of the claim or its complexity, the case may be heard in the High Court rather than the lower county court. The dentist does not usually attend this initial case management conference. The judge will seek to limit the issues at this conference and so will want to know if there are any areas of agreement between the parties. The courts now have fairly wide powers in how cases may be managed and so judges may make a variety of directions at this stage, including appointing a single expert, insisting on the experts meeting to narrow the issues, staying the case whilst a mediation takes place, etc. The courts will certainly seek to find ways of resolving disputes as early as possible. Generally at the end of the case management conference the times for exchanging lists of documents, witness statements and experts' reports before trial will be scheduled. The length and date of trial may also be fixed.

Pre-trial steps

Disclosure

The first stage is for both parties to exchange lists of relevant documents that they have in their possession that they must disclose to the other side. Generally these are clinical records (including radiographs, study models, laboratory sheets, etc.), correspondence, receipts for items of the special damages claims, etc. This step is to ensure that both parties have all the relevant information available to them which is pertinent to the issues in the case. Generally all the correspondence between a party and their solicitors, or advisers, attracts legal privilege; that is, it is not disclosed to the other side. Once an unprivileged document is enclosed in the list then the other party has the right to inspect it or request copies.

Witness statements, expert reports and schedule of special damages

The next stage, usually some months later, is for the parties to simultaneously exchange witness statements. Both the defendant and the claimant will be required to provide detailed witness statements, setting out their recollections, and statements from other witnesses such as dental surgery assistants, claimants' relations, etc. may also be produced.

Some months after exchange of witness statements the similar simultaneous exchange of expert reports takes place. This crucial step really enables each party to fully appraise the merits and weaknesses of their respective cases. This is usually the stage at which cases may settle if they have not already done so.

It is not generally possible to produce any evidence at court if it has not been exchanged in accordance with the court directions.

Near to trial the claimant will be required to serve an up-to-date schedule of special damages in order that the potential present value of the claim is clear. The defendant may subsequently serve a counter schedule if items claimed are in dispute.

Payment into court

At any stage, once proceedings have been issued, the defendant can make a payment into court[18] additionally, and similarly, to any previous offer to settle in the letter of response. The defendant pays into the court office the amount of compensation he/she is offering to settle the case and the claimant has 21 days to consider the payment. If the claimant chooses not to accept and subsequently succeeds and recovers more at trial, there is no problem. If, following refusal, the same or less in damages is subsequently recovered, then there is a considerable costs penalty in that the claimant is responsible for paying his/her own and the defendant's legal costs from 21 days after the payment was made despite the fact he/she eventually won the case. This costs penalty can effectively swallow up all the compensation.

Trial

The trial is heard by a judge alone who will not know if there has been any payment into court and nor will it be the same judge who dealt with previous case management issues. There is no jury and the court is open to the public and if the case is of local or national media interest, it may be reported by attending journalists. Both the defendant and claimant will be required to attend the trial and will usually be represented by a barrister with whom they will have met before to discuss and prepare the case. Both the claimant and defendant will be required to give evidence under oath and the evidence will usually entail reading out detailed witness statements. They will then be questioned by their own barrister in order to clarify any points (examined), questioned by the opposing party's barrister (cross-examined) and then finally asked further questions by their own barrister (re-examined) to clarify any matters arising from cross-examination. The court procedure is adversarial and is often not a comfortable experience for the defendant and claimant. Any other witnesses will then go through a similar procedure.

It is worth bearing in mind that usually a claimant will recall the events more clearly than the defendant. The defendant, who has his/her clinical notes to rely on, will see very many patients and so it may be very difficult to recall matters that are not accurately, and contemporaneously, recorded in the clinical records some years after the event. For this reason, at trial if there is a conflict regarding the events between the parties then the judge will normally prefer the claimant's recollection.

Experts will then similarly be examined, cross-examined and re-examined on their evidence regarding the clinical events and issues.

The judge may then ask questions of any of the witnesses to clarify matters and the barristers for both the dentist and claimant will make closing speeches. After the judge has heard all the evidence he/she will then proceed to give judgement. This may be given orally at the end of the case or may be provided in a written judgement in the weeks following the case. If either party is unhappy with the judgement then they are usually able to appeal against it if they so wish.

Payment of compensation and costs

Upon judgement if the claimant succeeds then compensation will be paid within a short period of time. Legal costs will then need to be paid by the losing party to the winning party. Sometimes the amount of costs will be agreed but often after a trial the court will formally assess the amount of reasonable costs which are to be paid.

Conclusion

It is impossible to be precise as to the likely course of events in any litigation and this chapter has only considered the major and more common features in cases which go to trial. There has not been the opportunity to examine the detailed law that can surround each stage and form the substance of substantial 'legal argument'. Each case differs on its own facts and will be progressed accordingly within the general framework discussed. If it is any consolation, only a very small number of all clinical negligence cases proceed to trial as the majority are settled out of court.

References and notes

1 Bartonshill Coal Co v McGuire [1858].
2 Bolam v Friern Hospital Management Committee [1957].
3 Bolam v Friern Hospital Management Committee [1957] as confirmed by Whitehouse v Jordan [1981].
4 Nettleship v Weston [1971]. *See also* Wilsher v Essex Health Authority [1988] regarding newly qualified practitioners.
5 Roe v Minister of Health [1954].
6 Bolitho v City and Hackney Health Authority [1998]; Hucks v Cole [1993].
7 Sale and Supply of Goods Act 1994.
8 Hotson v East Berkshire Area Health Authority [1987]; Kay v Ayrshire and Arran Health Board [1987].
9 Alcock v Chief Constable of South Yorkshire Police [1991].
10 Selvanayagam v University of West Indies [1983].
11 *See* Judicial Studies Board guidelines and Criminal Injuries Compensation Board guidelines on damages.
12 Appleton and others v Garrett [1997].
13 The Health Act 1999; General Dental Council (1997) *Maintaining Standards*. GDC, London.
14 Access to Justice Act 1999.
15 Data Protection Act 1998.
16 Clinical Negligence Protocol as set out in Civil Procedure Rules 1999, Section B.
17 Civil Procedure Rules 1999 Part 1, The overriding objective.
18 Civil Procedure Rules 1999 Part 36.
19 Civil Procedure Rules Part 35. *See also* associated practice direction.
20 CPR Rule 35 and associated practice direction; *see also* Lord Chancellor's Department Draft Code of Guidance for Experts under the Civil Procedure Rules 1999.
21 The Limitation Act 1980.
22 The Limitation Act 1980 section 33.
23 *See* Civil Procedure Rules 1999 Part 3 for courts' case management powers.

CHAPTER THIRTEEN

Legal considerations in Scotland

Helen Kaney

Have regard for your name, since it will remain for you longer than a great store of gold.

(The Apocrypha, *Ecclesiasticus* 41:12)

Introduction

The ethical obligations of dentists apply throughout the UK but there are some specific legal issues that relate only to Scotland.

The law of negligence

The law of negligence in Scotland is known as delict,[1] which compares with the English law of tort. Delict is part of the civil law and the commission of a delict is the breach of an obligation created by the law. It is the area of law that makes conduct of which the law would disapprove actionable in the civil courts, in that a pursuer (a patient) may allege negligence against a defender (a dentist) and claim damages for the resulting harm caused. There are differences between the English tort and the Scots law of delict, for example in the law relating to defamation, however '... in the most frequently litigated area, that of negligence, it cannot be said that the law is not now the same in both jurisdictions'.[2]

Negligence has been defined as: 'The omission to do something which a reasonable man would do; or, doing something which a reasonable man would not do'. This quote is taken from one of the most well-known cases in the law of negligence, Donoghue v Stevenson.[3] This case went to the House of Lords and established one of the basic principles of the law of negligence.

As an extension of the legal principles established in Donoghue v Stevenson, it has been clearly established in law that a doctor or dentist treating a patient owes that patient a duty of care, not to injure or harm them. This professional liability can occur by means of a legally binding contract, either verbal or written. However, the existence or absence of a contract does not preclude the existence of a duty arising from the law of negligence. In respect of medical or dental treatment, there may also be liability based on assault.[4] However, liability is usually in issue because of unintentional harm due to a lack of the care required by law, i.e. negligence.

There are very few cases in existence where dentists have been successfully sued in court.[5] However, there are cases involving doctors the legal principles of which apply equally to dentists. The test for medical negligence has been set out in two leading cases, one in Scotland and the other in England. The most famous Scottish medical case, which established the legal principles, was Hunter v Hanley.[6] In this case Lord President Clyde outlined a test to be used when trying to establish medical negligence. He said:

> First of all it must be proved that there is a usual and normal practice; secondly it must be proved that the defender has not adopted that practice; and thirdly (and this is of crucial importance) it must be established that the course the doctor adopted is one which no professional man of ordinary skill would have taken if he had been acting with ordinary care.

He further added:

> The true test for establishing negligence in diagnosis or treatment on the part of a doctor is whether he has been proved to be guilty of such failure as no doctor of ordinary skill would be guilty of if acting with ordinary care.

These Hunter v Hanley tests are essential in establishing medical or dental negligence in Scotland. When the standard of care provided is examined, it is also important to note that the courts will look at the knowledge and views of the profession at the date of the alleged breach of duty rather than at the date of the trial.[7]

The legal principles of Hunter v Hanley were two years later incorporated into a case in England, which established the Bolam test.[8] The case involving Mr Bolam found that in order to establish that a breach of clinical duty of care has occurred, the plaintiff[9] must show, to the satisfaction of the court, that what was done in the way of treatment did not correspond to that which a reasonable body of responsible medical opinion would accept as proper at the time of the incident.

In a Scottish case, Gordon v Wilson,[10] the Court of Session in Edinburgh held that where there were two differing bodies of medical opinion, which disagreed as to whether the conduct in question fell below the standard of care required, the court could not make a finding that the doctor had been negligent. We can see from this the 'tests are essentially the same in England and Scotland'.[11] However, as a result of the Hunter v Hanley tests, then if it is 'possible to find just one doctor (or dentist) whose opinion the court accept and who affirms that he or she would have followed the same course as the defender, then no matter how many contrary voices are heard, the pursuer will lose'.[12]

In the Bolitho case[13] the Bolam test was reaffirmed but it was stated that the opinion of the experts relied upon must be reasonable, responsible and logical and the court had the power to prefer one view to another.

Once it has been established that the standard of care provided fell below that required by law then the issue of causation must be considered. If after medical or dental treatment, someone is worse off than before they started, they still have to show that it was the dentist's fault that caused the harm suffered. In Kay's Tutor v Ayrshire and Arran Health Board[14] a medical claim was successfully defended on causation grounds.

The issues of duty of care, standard of care, breach of duty and causation are all individual hurdles which pursuers must clear in order to prove their case. The onus is on pursuers to prove their claim and the standard of proof is the civil standard, i.e. on the balance of probabilities.

The Scottish courts

Criminal courts

The district court is the lowest level of criminal court. The sheriff courts are the next level of courts and hear both criminal and civil cases, whereas the High Court of Justiciary is the highest level of criminal court. Appeals in criminal matters are to the High Court of Justiciary sitting as an appeal court. There is no appeal to the House of Lords in criminal matters.

Prosecution process

The prosecution of crime is almost exclusively the prerogative of the crown. The right to private prosecution still exists but is rarely invoked.[15] The Crown Office in Edinburgh is headed by the Lord Advocate and is responsible for the prosecution of all crime in Scotland. The Lord Advocate is assisted by the Solicitor General and 12 Advocates Depute, who conduct prosecutions in the High Court.

The Procurator Fiscal

The PF is the prosecutor in the sheriff and district courts. The office of the PF decides on whether or not prosecution is warranted, whether or not to take a case to trial and investigates all anaesthetic deaths. Recent high-profile investigations have occurred into deaths of children undergoing general anaesthesia in dental clinics.[16] It is possible that criminal charges could be brought against dentists in relation to their clinical work with patients, for example for failing to obtain consent to treatment, under the law of assault.

Criminal liability

Traditionally, in Scotland, the crime of assault required 'evil intent'. However, it has been argued that evil intent is not required, merely that it be a deliberate act. This means that a charge of assault could arise from a dentist–patient relationship, depending on the circumstances.[17] It is important to realise that there is an inter-relationship between the intention of the accused and the consent of the patient. Consent is no defence to a charge of assault in criminal law,[18] whereas it is a defence in civil law. In addition, the crime of causing real injury could be charged,[19] which requires recklessness as opposed to intent. Dental treatment, if sufficiently reckless, or indeed negligent treatment done intentionally, could be prosecuted under the criminal law in Scotland as its common law system is sufficiently flexible to adapt to new circumstances.[17]

Fatal accident inquiry

This is similar to a coroner's inquest in England and Wales. Investigations into a sudden or unexplained death are conducted in private by the Procurator Fiscal, who reports to the Crown Office with a view to instigating a FAI. This is a public inquiry and is advertised in the press a minimum of 21 days before the date on which it will be held in the sheriff court.[20]

Scottish civil courts

The sheriff courts are the lowest civil courts, whereas the Court of Session is the highest civil court based in Scotland. The House of Lords is the ultimate court of appeal in civil matters both in Scotland and the rest of the UK. However, the House of Lords has no jurisdiction to hear appeals for criminal cases arising in the Scottish courts.

Negligence claims in Scotland`

Patients who are intending to initiate an action for negligence will generally consult a solicitor. Dental records are requested[21] and the patient's solicitor will obtain a report from an appropriate expert on whether the standard of treatment provided has fallen below the standard required by law, i.e. the Hunter v Hanley tests. If the claim is against a GDP, then a GDP expert report should be obtained.[22]

The claim is intimated to the dental practitioner concerned or his/her defence organisation. At this stage, the dentist's defence organisation will investigate the matter, which may include the commission of their own expert report on breach of duty and causation issues and advice from their solicitors. The claim may be settled at this stage if there is obvious evidence that the case is indefensible.

Breach of contract

Litigation against a doctor or dentist is usually on the basis of negligence but could also be based on breach of contract. In this case, the Sale and Supply of Goods Act 1994 states that the treatment provided must be of 'satisfactory' quality, i.e. quality that would be acceptable to the reasonable patient (*see* Chapter 12).

> If it can be proved that the practitioner failed to fulfil his part of the bargain, a valid claim might arise. A dentist who undertook to fill a gap successfully ... might be liable if he failed. As with any suggested breach of contract, one of the major hurdles facing the pursuer is the need to prove the initial undertaking or promise.[12]

Litigation in Scotland

If agreement is not reached then court proceedings may be issued. Solicitors will be formally instructed by the dental defence organisation to act on behalf of the dental practitioner. The first stage is the formal serving of a writ[23] or summons on the defender or his/her legal representatives. These are the documents formally commencing court action and they include a statement of the allegations against the defender, a demand for reparation and an indication of the amount of compensation being sought. Following this a process of negotiation may ensue, defining the contested issues, and offers may be made to settle the claim.

If the claim is being defended then the defender's solicitors have 21 days from the serving of the writ to lodge a Notice of Intention to defend. This is lodged in the sheriff court and intimation is made to the pursuer or his/her representatives. Defences are lodged after a further four weeks, detailing what is admitted and what is denied. After further legal procedures, both sides advise whether they are ready to proceed to proof, i.e. civil trial.

When an action is being raised in the court of session, the first stage in the proceedings is to serve a summons on the defender. Defences are lodged and an adjustment roll is then opened for 12 weeks, which is an open record where written pleadings can be adjusted. If a case is going to proof (trial) it requires instruction of counsel, i.e. advocates who have rights of audience in the court of session,[24] whereas solicitors can appear in the sheriff court.

Trial is an adversarial process where the pursuer, defender and expert witnesses are required to give evidence in front of a sheriff or court of session judge sitting alone. Once the trial is complete, judgement is given and damages awarded, although appeal against the judgement is possible. Trial by jury in civil cases can only occur in the court of session but these are very rare.[25]

There is no financial limit to the amount of damages that can be awarded in the sheriff courts. However, raising an action in the court of session may be done if the matter is of particular complexity, e.g. involving a new legal argument or if English case law is relevant, and will undoubtedly result in a more high-profile case.

The pursuer must bring the action for alleged dental negligence within a three-year time limit,[26] which accords with the law in the rest of the UK. The three-year period begins to run on the date of the alleged negligent act in question or from the date of the patient's knowledge of the alleged negligent act. The courts also have discretion to admit a claim where it seems equitable or fair that it should do so.[27]

A comparison with England

In England the Civil Procedure Rules 1999 have resulted in much tighter deadlines for the investigation and handling of a claim than previously existed. These rules do not apply in Scotland, where up to a year may be an acceptable period of time for initial investigation of the claim. There is no equivalent to an offer to settle (*see* Chapter 12) in Scotland, but once court proceedings have commenced in Scotland, a defender can make an offer to tender. This is a formal offer in the judicial process, made by the defender to the pursuer to settle the action by payment of a specific sum together with expenses to the date of the tender. If the tender is not accepted and the court awards the pursuer the same or a lesser sum than that tendered, the pursuer will normally be found liable for any expenses incurred by the defender from the date of the tender. A defender may also make an offer to settle outwith the judicial process.

Damages in Scotland

The infringement of the right to bodily integrity, by the conduct of another, which is held to have been in breach of a legal duty, is remediable by an award of damages.[28] In Scotland the patient is made an award of solatium to compensate for their pain and suffering and patrimonial loss to compensate for their financial losses. Receipt of damages represents compensation for pain, suffering, injury to health, reduced life expectancy or death.[29] In fatal claims, the court allocates a proportion of the award for distress, grief and loss of society. Interest is awarded for the period from the date of the incident to the date of the decree[30] and deductions are made from the sum awarded for patrimonial loss for any benefits received under the Social Security (Recovery of Benefits) Regulations 1997.

Damages awarded to patients are increasing and Scottish courts take into account awards made by English courts in comparable cases and these can provide assistance in quantifying damages.[31] In general awards made in Scotland tend to be less than those in England; however, Scottish solicitors and advocates are increasingly likely to ask a trial judge to consider the level of damages awarded in English cases and award a comparable amount in Scotland.

Consent to treatment in Scotland

Ethical principles apply throughout the whole of the UK, governed by the General Dental Council. Individuals have the fundamental right not to have their bodily integrity violated. If treatment is provided without consent, then this will constitute both the crime of assault and an actionable civil wrong for which damages may be sought.

The legal age at which a person can consent to medical or dental treatment is 16 years.[33] In Scotland this is governed by Section 1(1)(b) of the Age of Legal Capacity (Scotland) Act 1991, which gives legal capacity to a person over 16 years to enter into a transaction, with transaction being defined to include 'the giving by a person of any consent having legal effect.' Consent to medical or dental treatment has legal effect, as it confers upon the doctor or dentist concerned a defence to an action for assault that the treatment would otherwise constitute.

For a child under 16, consent is governed in England and Wales by the decision in the Gillick case.[34] In Scotland the law is similar in that persons under 16 years can also consent to medical or dental treatment. The Age of Legal Capacity (Scotland) Act 1991 section 2(4) provides that:

> A person under the age of 16 years shall have the legal capacity to consent on his own behalf to any surgical, medical or dental procedure or treatment where, in the opinion of a qualified medical practitioner attending him, he is capable of understanding the nature and possible consequences of the procedure or treatment.

A child of any age can therefore give valid consent if he or she is considered by the practitioner to understand the nature of the proposed treatment. It has been argued that while the Act 'does not in its terms confer the right to refuse consent, the right to consent necessarily carries with it the right to refuse that consent'.[35] In this aspect, the law in Scotland arguably differs from that in England, although this has not been tested by the courts.

The capacity to consent under the 1991 Act is wide ranging, expressly covering both procedures and treatment and it 'therefore includes diagnostic procedures, experimental procedures, cosmetic surgery, donation of body tissue or organs and contraceptive or abortion advice and treatment'.[35]

For a child who does not have capacity to consent to treatment under the 1991 Act, the law is governed by the Children (Scotland) Act 1995.

Confidentiality

Ethical principles of confidentiality apply throughout the UK. The Age of Legal Capacity (Scotland) Act 1991 did not specify whether a child is entitled to confidentiality from a doctor or dentist; however, 'It is submitted that confidentiality is one of the passive rights that a child can be the holder of'.[35] The child's passive capacity to be the holder of rights is expressly preserved by section 1(3)(e) of the Act.

> It would be consistent with the policy of this Act . . . to hold that a child is entitled to confidentiality . . . when the child understands the nature and consequences of confidentiality, and wishes and expects it.[35]

There is therefore a duty of confidentiality to a child. However, there is also a duty to the parent in relation to consent, depending on the age of the child. Dentists are advised to counsel children and obtain their agreement to keeping the parent informed.

Practising in the NHS in Scotland

Dentists working in general dental practice must comply with the relevant regulations. These are the National Health (Scotland) Act 1978 and the National Health Service (General Dental Services) (Scotland) Regulations 1996 as amended. The NHS (GDS) (Scotland) Regulations 1996[36] detail the general arrangements for the provision of general dental services within the NHS. Schedule 1 to these regulations details the Terms of Service for dentists working in general dental practice.

Dentists working in general practice can work as assistants, associates or principals. Associates and practice owners apply to the relevant health board for inclusion in the dental list and are allocated a list number. This number is then used in all claims for payment from the Scottish Dental Practice Board via the health board. Although associates work in a practice owned by another dentist, they are actually principals in their own right, both in relation to the claiming of payment for work done in the NHS and also dento-legally.

Assistants, on the other hand, work on the same list number as the dentist employing them and are legally regarded as employees. The employing dentist is responsible to the SDPB for the acts and omissions of that assistant. While assistants should have their own professional indemnity cover, the employing dentist would be pursued in an action for negligence if they do not, even if he or she did not actually treat the patient. Indemnity cover is both an ethical[37] and a legal requirement.[38]

Health boards in Scotland

Scotland has 15 health boards and about 1850 dentists in general practice.[39]

Scottish Dental Practice Board

The Scottish Dental Practice Board in Edinburgh is the statutory body responsible for the authorisation of payments to dentists and for monitoring dental treatment. The Dental Practice Division (DPD) is the operational arm of the SDPB. One of its main roles is the authorisation of payments to GDPs through the processing of claim forms submitted by dentists. This payment system throws up a wealth of statistical information about the provision of general dental services in the NHS in Scotland. The DPD of the SDPB authorises the relevant health boards to pay dentists for the NHS work claimed. This information is then summarised in the annual practitioner profiles sent out to dentists.

Monitoring

Monitoring of the provision of dental services is done by the Scottish Dental Reference Service. Their function is to monitor the quality and probity of dental treatment by reviewing a sample of patients each year.

Where a potential breach of the Terms of Service is identified, the SDPB will refer the case to the appropriate Health Board for possible disciplinary action. If proven, the outcome of such a reference can be a referral to the General Dental Council, a withholding of remuneration or a period of prior approval. In some circumstances, the investigation by the health board and the DPD may result in a criminal prosecution.

NHS complaints procedures and disciplinary proceedings

NHS complaints procedures and disciplinary proceedings apply throughout the UK and there are no relevant differences relating to Scotland.

The Scottish Parliament and healthcare

The Scotland Act became law in November 1998. As part of the devolution settlement, the Scottish Executive, the First Minister and the new Scottish Parliament now have responsibility for devolved issues in Scotland such as health, housing and education. The NHS in Scotland has its own management executive.

However, regulation of the health professions currently regulated by Act of Parliament is a matter reserved to the UK Parliament under the Scotland Act 1998 and this includes the Dentists Act 1984. This means that the new Scottish Parliament has no power to amend the Dentists Act. This can only be done by Parliament in Westminster.

Conclusion

This chapter highlights the main differences in law that are relevant to the dental practitioner in Scotland. As already discussed, ethical considerations are the same as dentists practising elsewhere in the UK. Minor legal differences exist with regard to statutory authority for obtaining consent from young persons. However, procedural requirements are different from those in England, especially in view of the new Civil Procedure Rules 1999, which do not apply in Scotland.

In general, it can be said that patients are becoming more aware of the possibility of initiating a claim if treatment does not fulfil their expectations.

They are more questioning and less willing to accept any adverse consequence following treatment. Most claims are dropped or settled prior to litigation, but the stress involved for the practitioner concerned should not be underestimated. In all cases dentists are advised to consult their defence organisation for advice, support and assistance.

Acknowledgements

I would like to thank Dr Kevin Irvine and Alan J Mulrooney for their help in preparing this chapter.

References and notes

1   *Delinquo*, supine *delictum*, means 'to be lacking' or 'fail'. It was already used in classical Latin to mean 'fail in one's duty, offend'.
2   Stewart WJ (1998) *Delict* (3e). W Green and Son, London.
3   Donoghue v Stevenson [1932] *SC (HL)* 31.
4   In Scotland the term is 'assault', in England the term is 'battery'.
5   Appleton and others v Garrett [1997] *8 Med LR*.
6   Hunter v Hanley [1955] *SLT* 213.
7   Moynes v Lothian Health Board [1990] *SLT* 444.
8   Bolam v Friern Hospital Management Committee [1957] *2 All ER* 118.
9   Since the new Civil Procedure Rules in 1999, the plaintiff is now called the claimant. In Scotland the term is 'pursuer'.
10   Gordon v Wilson [1992] *SLT* 849.
11   Fulton Phillips A (1997) *Medical Negligence Law: seeking a balance*. Dartmouth.
12   Dickson RH (1997) *Medical and Dental Negligence*. Butterworths, London.
13   Bolitho v City and Hackney Health Authority [1997] *3 WLR* 1151.
14   Tutor v Ayrshire and Arran Health Board [1987] *SLT* 577.
15   *See* X v Sweeney and Another [1982] *SCCR* 509.
16   *Daily Mail*, 14 September 1999.
17   HMA v Duff [2000].
18   Smart v HMA [1975] *SLT* 65.
19   *See* Khaliq v HMA [1984] *SLT* 137.
20   *See* Fatal Accidents and Sudden Deaths Inquiry (Scotland) Act 1976 and Fatal Accident and Sudden Deaths Inquiry Procedure (Scotland) Rules 1977.
21   Data Protection Act 1998, formerly Access to Health Records Act 1990.
22   Scott v Highland HB OH, unreported 1981 and Aird v Ramsay Sh Crt, unreported 1984.
23   A writ is served if proceedings are being raised in the sheriff court, a summons if in the court of session.
24   Solicitor-advocates also have rights of audience in the higher courts.

25 Court of Session Act 1988.
26 Prescription and Limitation (Scotland) Act 1973 as amended.
27 Section 19A (1) of Prescription and Limitation (Scotland) Act 1973.
28 Damages (Scotland) Act 1976 and Damages (Scotland) Act 1993.
29 Damages (Scotland) Act 1993.
30 Interest on Damages (Scotland) Act 1971.
31 Allan v Scott [1972] *SC* 59.
32 www.gdc-uk.org
33 In England this is governed by the Family Law Reform Act 1969.
34 Gillick v West Norfolk and Wisbech Health Authority [1984] *QB* 581.
35 Norrie KM (1991) *The Age of Legal Capacity (Scotland) Act 1991.*
36 Statutory Instrument 1996 No. 177(S.14).
37 General Dental Council (1997) *Maintaining Standards*. GDC, London.
38 Health Act 1999.
39 Scottish Dental Practice Board Annual Report 1998/99.

CHAPTER FOURTEEN

Medical and dental research

David E Gibbons

If you steal from one author it's plagiarism, if you steal from many it's research.

(Wilson Mizner, *Alva Johnston: the legendary mizner*)

Advances in the treatment and care of patients proceed through medical and dental research. The pioneering work of dental and medical researchers, both clinical and non-clinical, provides the evidence base for clinicians, in collaboration with their patients, to choose the most beneficial and effective form of care for the patient's condition. However, the research process is open to abuse in many forms. This chapter will explore the ethical dilemmas raised by medical and dental research, as well as describing how these dilemmas have been addressed through codes of practice and policy. It commences with some historical and contemporary examples of abuses of research. Following this some key ethical principles are identified which form the basis of the ethical considerations raised by medical and dental research. Codes of practice for researchers will be discussed. Finally the implementation of codes of practice through research ethics committees will complete the chapter.

Introduction

Research ethics can be considered as 'the more or less deliberate and systematic consideration of moral problems arising in connection with the conduct and consequences of scientific research'.[1] It constitutes an important interface between science and society. Abuses of research take several forms. Research carried out on human beings without their consent or knowledge is a clear example of an abuse of the research process; for example, research carried out on prisoners of the Nazis. However, other examples include the Tuskegee Syphilis Study and the Contraceptive Study of San

Antonio[1] in which apparently uncomprehending, vulnerable or dependent subjects, minority groups or impoverished people were used as research subjects.

Perhaps the best example from dental research was the 'Vipeholm Study'[2] in which individuals with learning difficulties living in an institutionalised setting were divided up into groups, for the purpose of feeding them different diets in order to test the relative cariogenicity of the different regimes. Not only were the individuals not consenting to participate but they were not informed that they were participating in research and that a potential outcome for some was that they would have decayed teeth with attendant problems. Where, then, the duty of care of the researcher or the idea of doing no harm or at least that for any individual there should be net benefit of good over harm?

It should be clear that there is a need for a code of practice for research ethics such that individuals are not abused and participation in research is both voluntary and informed.

Key ethical principles

The key ethical principles[3] to be considered are:

- beneficence – doing good
- non-maleficence – not doing harm
- respect for autonomy
- justice, particularly distributive justice
- scope[4] – scope of application.

The development of codes of conduct: the ethics of research

The first generally accepted code of conduct for researchers was derived as a result of the Nuremberg experiences in 1948. It stated that:

- researchers' obligations to individual subjects were to be placed above obligations to the state
- the distinction between therapeutic and non-therapeutic research is taken to have moral implications

• the principle of informed consent for the subject is recognised as morally essential.

These principles were accepted and elaborated in the Declaration of Helsinki[5] which was adopted by the 18th World Medical Assembly held in that city. Subsequently these have been amended over the years and further refined, the most recent being at the 49th Assembly held in Edinburgh in October 2000. The basic premise is maintained that 'the health of a patient is a doctor's first consideration'. This is incorporated in the International Code of Medical Ethics: 'A physician should act only in the patient's interest when providing medical care, which might have the effect of weakening the physical and mental condition of the patient'.

Whilst the law is a set of rules supported by the power of the state with appropriate enforceable sanctions, ethics rests primarily on the voluntary actions of individuals informed by their own consciences derived from their own culture and life experiences. Nonetheless, as a healthcare professional it is important to have agreed professional codes. The World Medical Association[5] has prepared the following recommendations as a guide to every physician involved in biomedical research involving human subjects. They are kept under constant review. The standards as drafted are only guidelines for physicians all over the world. Physicians are, however, not relieved from the criminal, civil and ethical responsibilities under the law of their own countries.

Basic principles

1   Biomedical research involving human subjects must conform to generally accepted scientific principles and should be based on adequately performed laboratory and animal experimentation and on a thorough knowledge of the scientific literature.
2   The design and performance of each experimental procedure involving human subjects should be clearly formulated in an experimental protocol which should be transmitted for consideration, comment and guidance to a specially appointed committee independent of the investigator and the sponsor provided that this independent committee is in conformity with the laws and regulations of the country in which the research experiment is performed.
3   Biomedical research involving human subjects should be conducted only by scientifically qualified persons and under the supervision of a clinically competent medical person. The responsibility for the human

subject must always rest with a medically qualified person and never rest on the subject of the research, even though the subject has given his or her consent.

4 Biomedical research involving human subjects cannot legitimately be carried out unless the importance of the objective is in proportion to the inherent risk to the subject.

5 Every biomedical research project involving human subjects should be preceded by careful assessment of predictable risks in comparison with foreseeable benefits to the subject or to others. Concern for the interests of the subject must always prevail over the interests of science and society.

6 The right of the research subject to safeguard his or her integrity must always be respected. Every precaution should be taken to respect the privacy of the subject and to minimise the impact of the study on the subject's physical and mental integrity and on the personality of the subject.

7 Physicians should abstain from engaging in research projects involving human subjects unless they are satisfied that the hazards involved are believed to be predictable. Physicians should cease any investigation if the hazards are found to outweigh the potential benefits.

8 In publication of the results of his or her research, the physician is obliged to preserve the accuracy of the results. Reports of experimentation not in accordance with the principles laid down in this Declaration should not be accepted for publication.

9 In any research on human beings, each potential subject must be adequately informed of the aims, methods, anticipated benefits and potential hazards of the study and the discomfort it may entail. He or she should be informed that he or she is at liberty to abstain from participation in the study and that he or she is free to withdraw his or her consent to participation at any time. The physician should then obtain the subject's freely given informed consent, preferably in writing.

10 When obtaining informed consent for the research project the physician should be particularly cautious if the subject is in a dependent relationship to him or her or may consent under duress. In that case the informed consent should be obtained by a physician who is not engaged in the investigation and who is completely independent of this official relationship.

11 In case of legal incompetence, informed consent should be obtained from the legal guardian in accordance with national legislation. Where physical or mental incapacity makes it impossible to obtain informed consent, or when the subject is a minor, permission from the responsible relative replaces that of the subject in accordance with national legislation.

Whenever the minor child is in fact able to give consent, the minor's consent must be obtained in addition to the consent of the minor's legal guardian.

12 The research protocol should always contain a statement of the ethical considerations involved and should indicate that the principles enunciated in the present Declaration are complied with.

Medical research combined with professional care (clinical research)

1 In the treatment of the sick person, the physician must be free to use a new diagnostic and therapeutic measure, if in his or her judgement it offers hope of saving life, re-establishing health or alleviating suffering.

2 The potential benefits, hazards and discomfort of a new method should be weighed against the advantages of the best current diagnostic and therapeutic methods.

3 In any medical study, every patient – including those of a control group, if any – should be assured of the best proven diagnostic and therapeutic method. This does not exclude the use of inert placebo in studies where no proven diagnostic or therapeutic method exists.

4 The refusal of the patient to participate in a study must never interfere with the physician–patient relationship.

5 If the physician considers it essential not to obtain informed consent, the specific reasons for this proposal should be stated in the experimental protocol for transmission to the independent committee.

6 The physician can combine medical research with professional care, the objective being the acquisition of new medical knowledge, only to the extent that medical research is justified by its potential diagnostic or therapeutic value for the patient.

Non-therapeutic biomedical research involving human subjects (non-clinical biomedical research)

1 In the purely scientific application of medical research carried out on a human being, it is the duty of the physician to remain the protector of the life and health of that person on whom biomedical research is being carried out.

2   The subjects should be volunteers – either healthy persons or patients for whom the experimental design is not related to the patient's illness.

3   The investigator or the investigating team should discontinue the research if in his/her or their judgement it may, if continued, be harmful to the individual.

4   In research on man, the interest of science and society should never take precedence over considerations related to the well-being of the subject.

Research ethics committees: the professional and legal regulation of research

In the UK (Health Circular HSG (91)5) the Department of Health required district health authorities to set up local research ethics committees (LREC) or later through the NHS Executive, multicentre research ethics committees (MREC) for research being undertaken involving more than five LRECs. Although there is no legal obligation on a potential researcher to submit a protocol to an ethics committee for approval most funding bodies stipulate as a requirement that approval is gained. Researchers within the NHS would be denied access to patients, patient notes and samples without such approval. The authority of the ethics committee, however, is informal and extra-legal.[6]

The International Conference on Harmonisation (ICH) *Good Clinical Practice Guidelines* nonetheless places a central role on research ethics committees to ensure that the guidelines are observed. This is pivotal for any person or organisation wishing to obtain a product licence for a pharmaceutical product, as it is a legal requirement.

The role of a research ethics committee is to advise[6] and it does this by ensuring through a peer review process of lay and professional personnel that researchers address the issues in their protocol.

The Declaration of Helsinki recognised that there is a distinction between the ethics of clinical practice and that of biomedical research and as a result there is an order of priority between the two. The ethics of practice is basic to that of medical research. Informed consent and the duty of care become prerequisites of research involving human subjects or their identifiable records in order to respect their autonomy. The basis of this is that an adult or morally competent person has the right to restrict the access to information about them and how that information may be used.

Privacy is the freedom of the individual to pick and choose for him or herself the time, the circumstances under which, and most importantly the extent to which her or his attitude, belief, behaviour and opinions is to be shared or withheld from others.[7]

Thus others should not have the ability to cause pain or degradation to an individual (non-maleficence).

Confidentiality then refers to the way in which private information is managed. Research ethics should reflect the views of society and of researchers and is culturally based, with peer pressure (through the peer review process) being used to ensure the adoption of and adherence to certain methodologies or norms.

The law exerts its influence through the identified ethical procedures and rules it generates particularly in such areas as the following:

1   The protection of an individual's welfare:
    - by ensuring informed consent with regard to patient selection, randomisation, control groups and placebo
    - through the promotion of well-being
    - by peer review through an ethics committee
    - through the maintenance of confidentiality
    - by reviewing equity/non-discrimination through reviewing exclusions.

2   Promotion of research and protection of researchers and the maintenance of academic freedom.
3   Punishment of fraud and abuse, e.g.'plagiarism', when a large body of another's ideas are presented as one's own or deliberate reporting of facts that the researchers know to be unsubstantiated, or 'selective reporting', presenting only those observations which support the point being made or 'trimming' the observations which differ most from the average. Avoidance of waste of valuable public resources.
4   Compensation for injuries – redressing any harm caused by research.
5   Prevention of conflicts of interest such as that between proprietary interests and public responsibilities. The question to ask is who are the beneficiaries of the research?

As in other areas of practice it is important to maintain standards in ethical research and in so doing, protect participants from harm, protect their rights and provide reassurance to the public that this is done.

As with clinical care and consent to treatment it is important that individuals' capacity to make reasoned decisions is respected and that those whose capacity is impaired are protected. Choice should be informed and without bias or coercion. Participants should have adequate time to make an unpressured decision. Equally, those wishing to withdraw from research should be free to do so without the need for explanations or fear of their subsequent treatment or their relationship with the researcher or institution being adversely prejudiced. Clinical researchers have an ethical obligation to maximise benefits and minimise harm. The risks involved should be explained and there should be an equitable distribution of both harm and benefit.[8]

Medical or healthcare research may of course be conducted both on patients and on healthy people. In research in medical practice the intent is to benefit the individual patient (therapeutic) rather than to gain knowledge of general benefit, whilst medical research focuses on interventions which advance knowledge to benefit patients in general (non-therapeutic) and are unlikely to benefit the individual patient.[1] Equally, research may be observational, without any direct interference with the subject, e.g. by using records, or it could be intrusive (interfering with the subject).

Research and audit

Whilst the recognition of such classes of research might be illuminating it does not appear to inform the debate on the differences between research and audit. The following resumé proposed by the Manchester LREC does, however, help in this regard.

Similarities between medical research and medical audit

Both require good study design and may use similar methodologies, e.g. prospective, retrospective, survey sampling, questionnaire design and statistical analysis.

Differences between research and audit

- Research adds to the knowledge base, i.e. it provides the evidence with which clinical policy is developed while audit ensures that the knowledge base is used.
- Audit is intended to influence the activities of an individual or a team (i.e. carried out locally) while research attempts to influence medical practice as a whole.

- Audit never involves experiments on either patients or healthy volunteers, never involves completely new treatments, giving placebos or random allocation of treatment groups.
- Audit never involves disturbance to the patient beyond that required for normal clinical management.

The interface between research and audit

- As the basis of clinical research is clinical practice, there is a clear relation between research and audit.
- Research and audit have much to contribute to each other. Audit is the final step of a good clinical research programme, i.e. it is in series with research and not parallel to it.
- Good clinical audit is possible only when clinical interventions and innovations are based on good clinical practice.
- Audit may identify areas where further research is needed.
- The process of audit allows the dissemination of the findings of clinical research.
- Audit may provide data that researchers can use.

Research is concerned with discovering the right thing to do: audit with ensuring that it is done right.

Development of new drugs and other pharmacological products

Most development work on new drugs is *phased* in its progress towards introduction.[9]

Phase I trials are normally small scale where the drug, maybe following animal experimentation, is introduced into humans and drug dynamic and metabolic studies are undertaken. In the USA as there is no perceived benefit to the individual this is undertaken on volunteers whilst elsewhere it is usually undertaken with patients.

Phase II is where there is a clinical investigation using controlled clinical trials designed to test effectiveness and relative safety. It is normally conducted on a limited number of closely monitored patients.

Phase III clinical trials are implemented after the effectiveness has been established, at least to a given level, and designed to gather additional evidence of effectiveness for specific conditions and more precise definitions of drug-related adverse effects.

Phase IV is a post-marketing clinical trial to study the long-term effect on morbidity and mortality or in a patient population not adequately studied in the pre-marketing phase, e.g. children.

Some research is undertaken on animals and this also requires an ethical legislative framework. The UK Cruelty to Animals Act of 1876 is probably the oldest law in the world for the protection of animals. It provided an early legislative framework for what was deemed at the time to be acceptable and probably arose as a result of commonly held ethical views.

Nonetheless the ethical questions remain for constant review.

- Can we accept animal experiments?
- If yes, does the relative importance of the experiment justify the possible discomfort or suffering of the animal?
- Who is going to make this judgement?

The reader is invited to reflect upon these questions which are fundamental to so much that is carried on in the name of product research and development in both health and beauty care.

References and notes

1 Berg K and Tranoy KE (eds) (1982) *Research Ethics*. Liss, New York.
2 Gustaffson BE *et al.* (1954) The Vipeholm Dental Caries Study. The effect of different levels of carbohydrate intake on caries activity in 436 individuals observed for 5 years. *Acta Odont Scand.* 11: 232–64.
3 Beauchamp TL and Childress JF (1983) *Principles of Biomedical Ethics* (2e). Oxford University Press, Oxford.
4 Gillon R (1995) *Philosophical Medical Ethics*. John Wiley, Chichester.
5 World Medical Association (1964) *Declaration of Helsinki. Recommendations guiding physicians in biomedical research involving human subjects*. WMA, Helsinki.
6 *Manual for Research Ethics Committees* (5e). King's College, London.
7 Kelman HC (1977) Privacy and research with human beings. *J Soc.* 33: 169–95.
8 Consumers for Ethics in Research (2000) *Medical Research and You*. CERES, PO Box 1365, London N16 0BW.
9 Levine RJ (1986) *Ethics and Regulation of Clinical Research*. Urban and Schwarzenberg, Baltimore.

Index